HEALTHCARE NEXT

Real Lessons from the AI Frontlines

PublishU Ltd

www.PublishU.com

Acknowledgements

This book grew out of two decades of conversations with people on the frontlines of healthcare AI. Some of those conversations are threaded explicitly through these pages; many more shaped the thinking that produced them.

My thanks to **Dr Robert Lorenz, President of Cleveland Clinic London,** for the foreword and for the example his career sets. And to the leaders of health and social care systems I have had the privilege of working alongside—for the honest conversations about what it actually takes to make change stick.

At PublishU, my thanks to **Matt Bird** and the team for getting the thinking from manuscript to print.

To the clinicians, operators and patients whose stories appear here in composite form—your willingness to share the unvarnished version is what makes this book different from the conference circuit.

For **Indira, Aryana and Rohan**—the generation this book is trying to leave a better system to. And for **Shyamala**—co-architect of the life that makes any of it possible.

Contents

Foreword

I vividly recall my family's trips to our local bank as a young boy. I remember pulling up to the austere, granite walls, waiting patiently in the high-ceiling lobby in the queue for our turn with the teller and standing on tiptoes to peer over the marble countertop. I can even smell the distinct fragrance of the pages of my own small green bank account ledger, where I could read the credits and debits that my hard-earned allowance generated.

That was 40 years ago, and I have not waited in a bank lobby for decades. Our stately bank, a pillar of our small community, lies empty, its granite and marble accumulating dust. Instead, the same transactional capabilities are at my fingertips, instantaneous access, 24/7 and with a fraction of the effort, to a comparable explosion of financial options in our largely cashless, modern-day economy.

Yet as president of a newly-built hospital in the UK, I recently passed through our patient waiting room, with its traditional coffee station and used magazines, filled with patients waiting to be called in to see my doctor colleagues. You and I both know that just like my childhood banking memories, our patient waiting room days are numbered as well. We can already visualise the future of 24/7 access to expert medical opinion available in our palm, expanded in its optionality in ways that we never would have imagined. And we know that the change will happen in a fraction of the time that the banking industry took to evolve.

The clinical horizon is coming into view—artificial intelligence (AI) that reviews a complete medical history in seconds, diagnostic systems that outperform the best-trained radiologists, bedside care augmented by algorithms that never tire and never forget. Whether that future is 5 years away or 10, it is no longer hypothetical. And that is precisely the point.

Yet with all this certainty and belief in the monumental health care change to our near-term future, why is it that a health care leader like myself, leading a world-renowned hospital, has successfully implemented very little AI outside of ambient listening based on large language models to improve our current day hospital operations? The case for improved efficiencies and productivity could not be more profound as we approach the second-half of the decade. The average operating margin for United States hospitals is a non-sustainable 2.5%, with 40% of rural hospitals considered at risk of closure due to financial pressures and a full 50% of American hospitals operating in the red. At the same time, 50% of hospital professionals cite burnout as their number one workplace concern, stressed by the ever-increasing pressure of time-constraints, increasing responsibilities and decreased professional satisfaction.

As 'Healthcare Next' will demonstrate to its readers, the addressable gap is showing health care leaders how to embrace, successfully adopt and sustain this profound technology. The case is clear, and the tools are present, but due to the bewildering variety of "successful" pilots, the awesome power and limitless possibilities that the technology represents and our day-to-day focus on keeping our hospital ships afloat, both financially and figuratively, we are left as leaders —distracted and somewhat inexperienced—unsure where to begin.

In late 2024, I attended a dinner with Arvind Krishna, the CEO of IBM. Surely a technology company as steeped in innovation as IBM would have had a grand strategy as to how to implement AI in its own operational processes and throughout its new product offerings. But as Krishna tells the story, it could not have been further from the truth. The place IBM started was automated employment verification letters for employees for mortgage applications. He related how this mundane and rote task of matching employee employment history with the data specifically requested by the bank and how the computer could greatly enhance the productivity of the HR professionals through robotic process automation connecting the necessary databases. As the savings spoke for themselves through enhancing the HR department's efficiency, more and more tasks became automated. By concentrating on building data platforms and addressing manual back-office functions, IBM quickly compiled an operating system that had value internally, which could be prioritised externally to make IBM users more efficient at a lower cost. The imperative in health care to initiate a similar type of operational transformation could not be clearer. In this first playbook for operational leaders, Janahan Tharmaratnam draws on decades of experience across multiple continents and health systems to cut through the confusion, establish a common vocabulary and lower the barrier to adoption. He shows us how to evaluate, procure and deploy AI against the operational problems that matter most today while building the foundation for the clinical transformation that follows. The clinical future will come. But the operational present cannot wait.

I look forward to carrying these lessons forward in my own work, across the institutions I have the privilege to shape, and to seeing what becomes possible when adoption truly takes hold, at scale, where the rubber meets the road.

Robert R. Lorenz, MD, MBA

President, Cleveland Clinic London

United Kingdom, May 2026

Introduction

Can AI Make Health Care More Human, Not Less?

I have watched a $15 million AI investment fail to reach a single patient. I have sat with a daughter carrying her mother's medication list on her phone because two hospital systems, both running AI pilots, couldn't share a prescription. I have listened to a frontline nurse describe, with perfect calm, how she builds workarounds every shift for technology that was supposed to help her. These are not stories from the past. They happened over the past 12 months. And they keep me awake at night, not because I don't know the answer to whether AI can make health care more human but because I know we are writing that answer right now, with every procurement decision, every governance shortcut, every pilot signed off without a plan to scale.

I've spent two decades inside health care systems: the National Health Service's (NHS) fragmented complexity, Gulf state modernisation at speed, North American health systems navigating the brutal gap between quality and access. I've sat in boardrooms where executives applaud AI pilots that will never scale. I've watched brilliant technology die in the gap between demonstration and deployment. I've seen vendors sell futures while frontline staff navigate systems that don't talk to each other. This book is what I wish existed when I started. Not a hymn to the technology, not a warning against it. A practitioner's honest account of what works, what fails and, most importantly, why.

The Paradox We Face

Here is what we know. Between 80% and 92% of health care AI pilots fail to scale beyond their initial deployment. Only 5% demonstrate calculable return on investment (ROI). Most organisations cite integration with existing electronic medical records as their primary barrier. The gap between vendor promise and production reality is vast, expensive and entirely predictable to anyone who has been on the ground.

The NHS's National Programme for IT, the largest civilian IT programme ever attempted, consumed £12.7 billion and was eventually broken apart after years of delays, vendor exits and limited clinical adoption. Dermatology AI tools that performed impressively in development datasets saw accuracy fall by up to a third when tested in diverse, real-world clinical settings. These aren't cautionary outliers. They're the pattern.

> And yet. Transformation is coming—faster than most health care leaders are prepared for.

Estonia has achieved 99% health data digitisation with patient-controlled records. Kaiser Permanente's ambient documentation programme returned 15,791 hours—seven working years of clinical time—to patient care. India created 730 million digital health accounts in three years. Foundation models that were science fiction in 2023 are being deployed clinically today.

The technology works when the foundations exist to support it. That's the whole argument. We have a two-to-three-year window, not to chase every trend but to build the infrastructure, governance and workforce capability that will determine whether AI makes health care more human or less.

Meet Samantha

Throughout this book, you'll follow Samantha. Not because her story is unique but precisely because it isn't.

Samantha is a 45-year-old NHS operations director with 20 years' experience in health care. She knows the system from the inside: the budget meetings, the strategy documents, the pilots that launch with great fanfare and quietly disappear when the champion moves on.

Eighteen months ago, her 74-year-old mother, Margaret, was diagnosed with vascular dementia and early heart failure. Now Samantha experiences the system she helped build from the other side. She juggles four patient portals to book appointments. She maintains her own spreadsheet of her mother's medications because the systems don't share data. She has become her mother's integration layer—the human middleware connecting fragments that technology should have connected years ago.

She sits in board meetings where executives celebrate the trust's "AI-powered care coordination platform". Under the table, her phone shows four disconnected portals. The platform they're celebrating has never touched her mother's care.

Samantha is exhausted. Frustrated. And still, despite everything she knows about how systems fail, hopeful. Because she's also seen the nurse who had time to hold her mother's hand while an ambient documentation system handled the charting. She's seen what connected infrastructure looks like when someone bothers to build it.

She knows change is possible. She's just not sure we're choosing to create it.

Samantha's journey is this book's spine. Her dual perspective—professional insider and exhausted family caregiver—is the lens through which we'll examine every technology, every trade-off, every choice.

The Flywheel

Here is the mental model I want you to carry through everything that follows:

In a flywheel, every rotation reinforces the next. Initial effort is high. The wheel resists. But once it starts turning, momentum builds. Each rotation becomes easier. Energy compounds.

Health care AI works exactly the same way when it works at all. Clinician adoption leads to better patient outcomes. Better outcomes build trust. Trust enables data sharing. Better data improves AI performance. Better AI makes clinician adoption easier. Round again. Faster. Building momentum.

But most organisations never get the flywheel spinning. They push hard on one spoke—usually the technology—and wonder why nothing moves. They don't realise the wheel is stuck because of friction elsewhere: poor data quality, fragmented systems, clinicians who don't trust the recommendations, governance structures that paralyse rather than enable.

Throughout this book, ask yourself, "Where is the flywheel stuck in my organisation? What's creating friction? What's the first push that gets it moving?" Because transformation isn't about algorithmic sophistication. It's about removing friction and building momentum, then letting the systems natural dynamics do the rest.

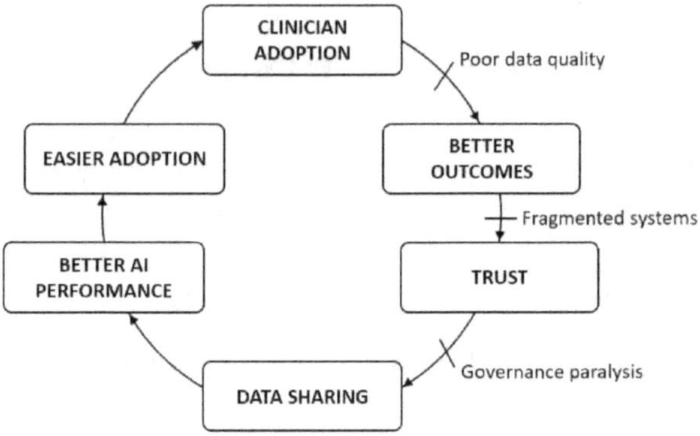

Figure 1. The health care AI flywheel—from initial push through self-sustaining momentum. Every rotation reinforces the next. Friction at any spoke—data quality, fragmented systems, governance paralysis—stops the whole wheel.

Three Things to Remember

If nothing else, carry these three principles:

1. Clarity before capability

   You cannot build what you do not understand. The organisations that succeed cut through vendor hype, establish shared vocabulary and confront uncomfortable truths before writing cheques. Those that fail chase capabilities before they know what problem they're solving.

2. Connection before intelligence

   AI can only care for what it can see. The most sophisticated algorithm is worthless if it can't access the data it needs, integrate with the systems clinicians use or connect information across care boundaries. The boring infrastructure work nobody wants to fund? That's what makes or breaks AI in health care.

3. Systems before showcases

   Patients live in systems, not pilots. The pilot that works in a controlled environment with dedicated support tells you almost nothing about whether the solution will work in production. Health care doesn't need more impressive demonstrations. It needs transformation that reaches every patient, survives when champions leave and compounds over time.

What's Possible

Before we get into the hard work, let me show you what's already operational.

In Estonia, an emergency department physician sees a patient's complete medical history the moment they arrive. No phone calls. No faxed records. X-Road infrastructure connects everything. Every citizen controls their own records. This isn't a vision document; it has been running since 2008. At Kaiser Permanente, Dr Hassan closes her laptop. Her clinical note is already drafted. Three minutes to review instead of 15 to document. The time she saved she spent with her patient. In rural India, a farmer creates his Ayushman Bharat digital health account—14 digits connecting identity to medical history, accessible wherever he seeks care. Seven hundred thirty million accounts. Created in three years.

The question isn't whether this transformation is possible. It's whether your organisation will prepare for it or watch others achieve it while you remain stuck explaining why the integration work is too complex to start.

What This Book Is and Isn't

This is a practitioner's book. The frameworks, questions and patterns here come from two decades of frontline work across health systems in six countries. It isn't theory dressed up as experience. It's what I've seen work, what I've watched fail and what I've learnt to distinguish between the two.

This book will be updated annually. This field moves too fast for any single edition to be definitive. What I'm committing to is honest, current guidance, not a static artefact.

This book is neither a technical manual for data scientists nor a comprehensive survey of every AI application in health care; nor is it neutral on whether AI transformation can be done well. It can. The question is whether we choose to do it that way.

How to Read This Book

Board members and executives trying to make sense of AI proposals: Start with Part I, Seeing Clearly. These three chapters will help you separate genuine capability from sophisticated marketing.

Leaders responsible for implementation who need practical frameworks: Go to Part II, Building Wisely. Infrastructure, integration, workforce—the things that actually determine whether technology reaches patients.

Those setting strategy and governance: Part III, Leading Forward, addresses value assessment, trust architecture and how to prepare for what's coming next, including agentic AI systems that are already in early deployment.

Clinicians wondering how AI will reshape your work: The chapters on augmentation and workforce address your questions directly without the usual techno-optimism or unnecessary alarm.

Aspiring leaders building careers in health care transformation: Read the whole thing. The vocabulary, frameworks and case studies here are what distinguish the people who talk about AI transformation from the ones who actually deliver it.

A Note on Evidence

I've tried to be honest about what we can prove, what we believe and what we don't yet know. The research base for AI in health care is growing but still thin. Most validation studies measure diagnostic accuracy, not patient outcomes. Most business cases rest on projections, not proof. Most success stories come from controlled pilots, not scaled implementations.

This book doesn't hide those gaps. It confronts them because the leaders I respect most are the ones who make decisions with intellectual honesty rather than optimistic projection, and they deserve a book written in the same spirit.

The Choice We Face

Can AI make health care more human, not less?

The answer isn't predetermined. It depends on choices we make every day about procurement, governance, what we measure, what we value and who we believe when they tell us something is working.

We can choose to chase every trend, fund impressive pilots that never scale and optimise for metrics that have nothing to do with patient well-being. That path leads to more fragmentation, more clinician burnout, more families navigating systems that AI was supposed to fix. Or we can choose clarity. Connection. Systems over showcases. We can demand evidence, build infrastructure, develop our people and keep the human—patient, clinician, family member—at the centre of every decision.

Samantha is in the garden with her mother. Margaret is having a good day; she's lucid, present and asking questions. "Will it get better?" she asks. "The health care?"

Samantha doesn't know how to answer. But by the end of this book, she will. And so will you.

Not because I have all the answers. Because I'll show you which questions to ask, what evidence to demand and what choices will shape whether AI makes health care more human or less.

The next two to three years will decide. Let's make sure we get them right.

PART I: SEEING CLEARLY

Chapter 1
The Hype Hangover

What the Frontlines Actually Reveal

Key message: Most of what you've heard about AI in health care is mixed, biased and often wrong. Here's what years on the frontlines actually reveal about the gap between promise and delivery and what to do about it.

If You Read Nothing Else, Remember These Five Things

1. Four out of five health care AI pilots fail to scale.

   The gap between vendor promise and production delivery is vast, expensive and predictable. Integration complexity, champion dependency and funding gaps kill more projects than technical failures ever will.

2. Success looks different than the conferences suggest.

   Microsoft's Nuance DAX Copilot took four-plus years to get right through relentless iteration. Kaiser Permanente's ambient documentation succeeded because they treated integration as the hard work, funded realistically and measured what mattered: clinician well-being, not algorithmic accuracy.

3. External validation is non-negotiable.

   Internal testing proves nothing about real-world performance. Dermatology AI showing 88 – 94% accuracy internally dropped to 56 – 67% externally. Some systems performed at random chance on darker skin tones. If vendors can't show external validation in populations like yours, you're their experiment.

4. "AI-ready" is organisational, not technical.

   Data quality matters, but governance, change management capacity, clinical engagement and leadership commitment determine success more than any algorithm. Most organisations overestimate their readiness by years.

5. Four questions cut through any vendor presentation.

   Has this been externally validated in settings like ours? What's the integration plan, not after deployment but before? Who owns ongoing maintenance when the champion leaves? What's the funding path from innovation budget to operational budget? If vendors can't answer these clearly, walk away.

Opening

The Board Meeting

The chief digital officer (CDO) advances to the next slide. "AI-Powered Care Coordination Platform: Year One Success." The boardroom screen fills with metrics—efficiency gains trending upward, user testimonials in carefully chosen quotes, a pilot showing promise.

Samantha sits three seats down, her phone hidden under the table. She's trying to book a follow-up appointment for her mother. Portal one: GP surgery. Portal two: hospital Electronic Patient Record (EPR). Portal three: memory clinic. Portal four: cardiac monitoring. None of them talk to each other. The memory clinic can't see last week's cardiology notes. The GP has no visibility of the medication change made during Margaret's last admission.

"Our AI platform is transforming patient care through intelligent coordination..." The executives nod. One asks about scaling to other pathways. Another about the business case for expansion.

Nobody mentions that the celebrated platform serves exactly one clinical pathway—diabetes—and has never touched 92% of the trust's patients.

Including her mother.

Samantha closes her phone. Returns it to her bag. She's not sure what she would say or whether anyone wants to hear it. The gap between the slides and Margaret's reality has become unbearable. But this is a board meeting celebrating success. This is not the moment for uncomfortable truths.

"With this foundation, we're positioned to expand AI across all our care pathways." Applause. The finance director asks about next year's budget. The meeting moves on.

Samantha makes a note in her planner: :Call GP about medication reconciliation. Again."

Field Lesson 1: The Promise-Reality Gap

The gap between what vendors promise and what health care actually gets is where most AI initiatives die. Not because the technology fails, though sometimes it does, but because the organisations deploying it don't fully understand what they're buying or what it takes to make it work.

Learning from Microsoft-Nuance: Iteration, Not Revolution

In 2020, Microsoft acquired Nuance Communications for $19.7 billion. They weren't buying a product; they were buying decades of health care expertise, established clinical relationships and the institutional knowledge of what it actually takes to get clinicians to change how they work. The story of DAX Copilot is worth understanding in detail because it demonstrates something the hype cycle consistently obscures: Successful health care AI is a long game.

The early iteration required four-hour turnaround times with human reviewers checking every AI-generated note. Clinicians recorded encounters, uploaded them and waited. It worked, but it wasn't the painless transformation the demos suggested.

What changed wasn't primarily the technology. Microsoft was humble enough to let Nuance lead. They embedded teams in hospitals. They listened to physicians saying, "This almost works, but..." The breakthrough came from deep integration with Epic (one of the leading Electronic Medical Record solutions), not surface-level connection but embedded workflow integration that let clinicians record encounters and review AI-generated notes without ever leaving the system they already used. Deployment time fell from 18 months to under six months. By 2024, over 600,000 clinicians worldwide were using Dragon Medical One solutions.

A 2024 survey of 879 clinicians across 340 organisations found five minutes saved per encounter, 70% reduction in feelings of burnout and fatigue and 84 – 88% reporting positive experiences. The Department of Veterans Affairs ran a 120-day competition involving 150 companies and selected DAX Copilot. Dr Christy Chan at Overlake described the change plainly: "I finally have weekends back." The lesson isn't that Microsoft's technology was special. It's that they treated the clinical integration problem, not the algorithm, as the real challenge. That distinction separates deployments that scale from those that don't.

The AI Washing Problem

The success of solutions like DAX stands in sharp contrast to most of what gets marketed as AI in health care. A 2019 survey found that 40% of European startups classified as AI companies didn't use artificial intelligence in any material way. By 2024, only approximately 10% of health care solutions marketed as AI met technical definitions of machine learning. The rest are rules-based automation from the 1990s wearing new branding.

This matters more than it might seem. Rules-based systems do exactly what they're programmed to do. They don't adapt. They can't handle cases that fall outside pre-defined parameters. When leaders expect the adaptability of machine learning but deploy rule-based rigidity, disappointment is structurally guaranteed. The vocabulary trap compounds the problem; organisations that conflate automation, analytics, machine learning and generative AI give vendors cover to hide limitations behind jargon.

The correction is simple, but it requires confidence to apply: Demand technical clarity before procurement. Ask vendors directly, "Is this machine learning or rules-based automation?" If they can't answer clearly, they're not ready. And neither are you.

What "AI-Ready" Actually Means

Most organisations overestimate their readiness for AI deployment. They focus on data quality, which matters, but underestimate the organisational, cultural and governance gaps that ultimately determine whether any implementation succeeds.

Structured data in electronic records represents only 20 – 30% of clinical information. The rest lives in free-text notes, scanned documents, images and conversations that were never documented. Even the structured data has problems: missing values, inconsistent coding, documentation quality that varies by clinician, temporal misalignment where diagnosis codes get entered after treatment has already begun. AI built on this foundation sees a partial picture at best.

But data quality, while necessary, is not sufficient. Organisations also need governance structures that can actually make decisions: who approves deployment, who monitors performance, who decides when to retrain or retire an algorithm. They need change management capacity that most teams underestimate by a factor of three. They need clinical champions who understand the technology and will genuinely advocate for it, not just tolerate it. And they need leadership commitment measured not in rhetoric but in resources, patience for a two-to-three-year journey and willingness to make hard calls when initial results disappoint.

"AI-ready" means the organisation is ready. Not just the technology.

Field Lesson 2: Why Pilots Don't Scale

The 80 – 92% pilot failure rate is health care AI's open secret. These projects don't succeed more slowly than hoped. They fail. They disappear from roadmaps. A 2024 survey found that only 6% of health systems successfully scaled generative AI beyond pilot stage. The rest are stuck in what I call pilot purgatory, celebrating demonstrations while patients experience fragmented care.

The Integration Cliff

Pilots work in controlled environments. There's a dedicated project team, flexible workflows, a data scientist sitting with clinicians solving problems in real time. Everyone involved wants the pilot to succeed and works around obstacles to make it happen.

Production is different. Production requires integration with systems that weren't designed to work together—the Electronic Medical Record (EMR) storing data in proprietary formats, the departmental systems using different patient identifiers, the laboratory information system that won't expose its API for security reasons, the radiology Picture Archiving and Communication System (PACS) that predates modern integration standards. Each connection requires technical work, governance approval, workflow redesign, training and ongoing maintenance. The total effort typically exceeds the effort required to build the AI itself by a factor of three to five. Vendors don't mention this in business cases. Project teams discover it mid-implementation. By then, the budget is committed.

The UK's NPfIT Lesson

The NHS's National Programme for IT (NPfIT) set out to build something no country (with a legacy and history like the NHS) had attempted: a fully integrated national health technology infrastructure. The ambition was exactly right. But the programme demonstrated that without clinical engagement, integration planning and the ability to adapt to local realities, even the best-funded programmes struggle to deliver lasting change. The lesson isn't about one programme. It's about a pattern that repeats wherever technical capability moves faster than organisational readiness.

The Champion Dependency

Almost every successful AI pilot has a champion—someone passionate, technically capable, politically savvy, willing to work around obstacles. They make the pilot succeed through force of will. Then they get promoted, are recruited elsewhere, burn out or move to the next exciting project. The pilot dies. Because the pilot succeeded through individual heroism, not institutional capability. The processes weren't documented. The workflows weren't standardised. The governance wasn't embedded. When the champion leaves, nobody else knows how to keep it working. Sustainable implementation requires standard processes that don't need heroes, documented workflows that new staff can follow and governance integrated into existing structures—not innovation budgets, but operational ones.

The Funding Gap

Innovation funding for pilots comes from different budgets than operational funding for scaled solutions. This gap kills more projects than technical failures. When the pilot shows promise and the champion requests operational funding, the finance department asks for ROI proof at scale. The champion can't provide it; that's what scaling is supposed to produce. Finance declines. The pilot dies. No one marks it as a failure. It simply stops appearing in the roadmap.

There is no clean answer to this problem. But ignoring it guarantees pilot purgatory. The organisations that navigate it successfully treat funding pathway as a design question, decided before the pilot begins, not after it succeeds.

Field Lesson 3: The Validation Question

External validation is where vendor claims meet reality. It is also where most AI solutions fail.

The Dermatology Story

Area under the curve (AUC) measures how well an algorithm distinguishes between conditions, where 1.0 is perfect and 0.5 is random chance. Scores above 0.85 typically appear in vendor presentations as evidence of clinical-grade performance.

Internal accuracy claims for dermatology AI systems in 2020 – 2022 were compelling: 88 – 94% AUC for skin cancer detection, published in leading journals, vendors announcing clinical deployment. Everything looked ready.

Then came external validation. A 2022 study in Science Advances[1] tested leading systems on a curated, diverse clinical image set. Performance dropped 27 – 36 percentage points, from 88 – 94% AUC to 56 – 67%. Systems that performed excellently in controlled testing failed in real clinical practice.

The equity dimension was worse. DeepDerm performed at random chance—AUC 0.50—on dark skin compared to 0.61 on light skin. The AI could not reliably detect melanoma in the populations where late diagnosis is most common and outcomes worst. A 2022 JMIR Dermatology study identified the root cause: Dark skin images represent only 4 – 18% of images in dermatology training datasets. The AI learnt what it was taught. It was taught with biased data.[2]

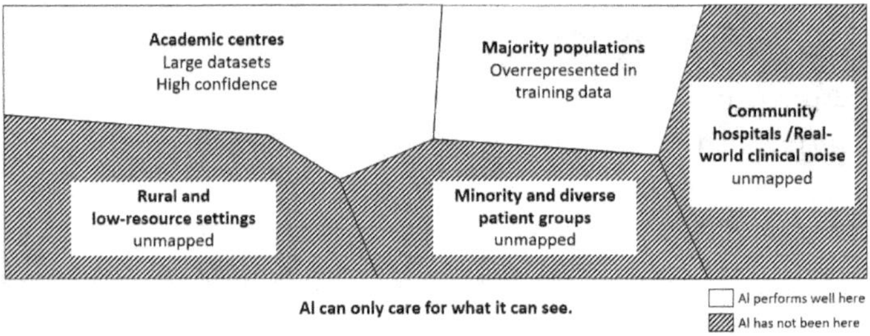

Figure 2. AI can only care for what it can see. Three zones remain unmapped.

The positive note, and there is one, is that the problem is solvable. When systems were fine-tuned on diverse datasets, the performance gap closed. A 2022 study in the Science Advances showed systems trained on adequately representative data performing comparably across all populations.[3] The lesson isn't that dermatology AI doesn't work. It's that internal testing tells you the algorithm works in controlled conditions and nothing more. External validation tells you whether it works for your patients. Demand it.

Field Lesson 4: What Success Actually Looks Like

Not all health care AI fails. Some succeeds but for reasons that have almost nothing to do with algorithmic sophistication.

Kaiser Permanente's Ambient Documentation

In 2023, The Permanente Medical Group in Northern California piloted Nabla's ambient documentation technology with 10,000 physicians. Careful, phased, with comprehensive quality checks. By August 2024, Kaiser expanded to Abridge's system across 24,600 physicians, 40 hospitals and over 600 medical offices across eight states. By early 2025, usage had exceeded 2.5 million patient encounters.

The outcomes: 15,791 hours of documentation time saved, approximately seven working years of clinical time returned to patient care. 84 – 88% of clinicians reporting positive experiences. Patients reporting that their physicians were more present and attentive during appointments. Clinician retention improving in an era defined by burnout and resignation.

Why did it scale when most don't? Kaiser treated integration as the hard work, not the afterthought. They integrated directly with Epic before widespread deployment. They phased the rollout deliberately, letting each stage inform the next. They measured what executives and boards actually cared about:

workforce sustainability and patient experience rather than algorithmic accuracy. They funded for scale from the start, with operational budgets built into annual planning. And their governance accelerated deployment rather than blocking it.

> "Abridge's advanced technology supports our doctors' well-being by reducing the documentation burden, which helps the physician to be more focused on the needs of the patient and their family."
>
> —Dr Brian Hoberman, CIO, The Permanente Medical Group

The success wasn't about finding the best algorithm. It was about treating every non-algorithm challenge—integration, funding, governance, measurement—as seriously as the technology itself.

Estonia: Infrastructure First

While Kaiser demonstrates AI deployment done well, Estonia demonstrates what happens when you build the foundation before the applications.

Since 2008, Estonia has built what other nations now reference as the benchmark: 99% of health data digitised, ranked first globally in the 2024 Digital Health Index, every citizen controlling their own records. The foundation isn't an AI system. It's X-

Road—a secure data exchange layer connecting all government and health care systems, built as national infrastructure, not a health care-specific project.

What X-Road enables in practice: An emergency physician sees a patient's complete medical history instantly. No phone calls. No faxed records. Ambulance crews access patient records en route. Specialists see the complete picture regardless of where previous care occurred. Patients log in to one portal and see everything including who accessed their data and when.

Why it succeeded where NPfIT failed: X-Road was operational before health care applications were built. Citizens control permissions and trust the system because of it. The investment was sustained over 16-plus years, not a three-year project hoping for political continuity. Even during construction, X-Road enabled incremental services; infrastructure investment without visible quarterly value typically means you're building the wrong thing.

Context matters. What works for 1.3 million people is not automatically transferable to 67 million or 330 million. But the principle translates: No amount of algorithmic sophistication overcomes fragmented infrastructure. Estonia built the foundation. Everything else became easier.

Framework Close: Four Questions Before Your Next AI Decision

Before approving any AI procurement, deployment or scaling decision, get clear answers to these four questions. If you can't, you're not ready to proceed.

1. Has this been externally validated in settings like ours?

   Internal testing proves the algorithm works in one environment. External validation proves it generalises. Demand evidence from settings with similar populations, similar workflows, similar data quality. If the vendor can't provide it, you're their external validation experiment. Decide consciously whether you're comfortable with that role.

2. What is the integration plan—before deployment, not after?

   Integration determines whether AI gets used. Demand detailed integration plans before procurement: which systems, which APIs, which workflows, which training, which governance approvals. If the vendor says they'll figure it out during implementation, they're not ready. And neither are you.

3. Who owns this when the champion leaves?

   Sustainable implementations don't depend on heroes. Before you start, ask who monitors ongoing performance. Who handles algorithm drift? Who provides support when the implementation team moves to the next project? If ownership isn't clear before deployment, the system won't survive the first staff transition.

4. What is the funding path from innovation to operations?

   Pilots need innovation funding. Scale needs operational funding. The gap between these kills most implementations. Map the entire funding journey before the pilot begins: innovation phase, scale phase, operational phase and who makes the decision to move between each. If the path isn't clear, you're building something that won't scale.

Back to Samantha

Dr Rahman used to dread his morning ECG queue. Forty to 60 flags, every day. "Anomaly detected, confidence 87%." "Irregular pattern identified, confidence 92%." No context. No explanation of clinical significance. No indication of urgency. He'd work through them during his lunch break, most turning out to be artefact—patient movement, electrode placement, normal variants the algorithm hadn't learnt to recognise. After six months, he stopped trusting the system. He'd click "acknowledge" without detailed review. If something was truly urgent, the nurses would page him. Then someone asked what he actually needed to see.

Three months after the board meeting, Samantha accompanies her mother to cardiology. Dr Rahman opens his laptop and explains what the system is showing now.

"Used to just say 'anomaly detected, 87% confidence.' I had no idea what that meant. Someone finally asked us what we needed to see. We told them: what changed, what it might mean, what we should consider. They rebuilt the interface. Took six months. Now I trust it." —Dr Rahman

"What made the difference?"

"They stopped trying to impress us with the algorithm. Started trying to help us care for patients."

Samantha makes a note. That's the pattern. Not the sophistication of the technology. The humility to ask what clinicians actually need and the discipline to build it.

Remember the Five Things

These aren't five separate lessons. They're a connected system, and the connection matters.

The 80 – 92% failure rate exists because organisations skip the hard questions. They don't demand external validation, so they deploy systems that work in controlled settings and fail in the real world. They don't plan for integration, so champions compensate through heroics that don't survive their departure.

They don't map funding paths, so pilots die in the gap between innovation and operations. They don't assess organisational readiness honestly, so governance paralysis, poor data quality and clinical resistance kill even good technology.

Microsoft-Nuance and Kaiser Permanente succeeded because they understood this. External validation in diverse settings before scale. Integration designed before deployment, not retrofitted after. Operational funding planned from the start. Organisational readiness built through genuine clinical engagement, real governance and leadership commitment measured in years, not announcements.

Most AI pilots will fail to scale.

Plan for integration complexity, champion dependency and funding gaps from day one. Don't assume your pilot will be the exception. Microsoft-Nuance took four years of iteration. Kaiser succeeded because they planned for the hard work. So should you.

Study the successes more carefully than the failures.

Microsoft didn't waltz into health care and dominate with algorithms. They bought expertise, listened to clinicians, integrated deeply with Epic and iterated relentlessly. Kaiser didn't deploy to 24,600 physicians overnight. Both measured what mattered: clinician well-being and patient experience, not accuracy metrics.

External validation is your insurance policy.

Dermatology AI looked perfect internally then dropped 30+ percentage points in diverse clinical settings. Internal testing tells you the algorithm works under controlled conditions. External validation tells you whether it works for your patients. Demand it. If vendors can't provide it, you're their experiment.

Organisational readiness matters more than data readiness.

Fix your data, yes. But also fix your governance, your change management, your clinical engagement, your leadership commitment. The failing organisations aren't primarily those with messy data; they're those without the organisational muscle to deploy anything successfully. AI just exposes the gaps that already existed.

Ask the four questions before every procurement decision.

External validation in settings like ours. Integration plan before commitment. Ownership after the champion leaves. Funding path from innovation to operations. If you can't get clear answers, you don't have enough information to proceed.

The gap between hype and reality isn't closing on its own. But it can be navigated. Organisations that demand clarity, plan for integration, build institutional capability and fund realistically are succeeding. Those that chase trends, celebrate pilots and assume scale will sort itself out are filling the pilot graveyard.

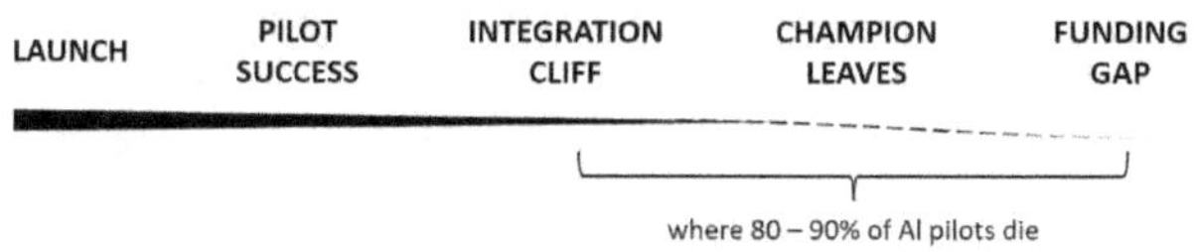

Figure 3. The pilot graveyard—where 80 – 92% of health care AI pilots fail to scale. Pilot success is not scale. The failure cascade begins at integration cliff, accelerates when champions leave and ends at the funding gap.

Samantha leaves the cardiology appointment and walks to her car. For the first time in 18 months, she didn't have to explain to a specialist what medications her mother was taking. Dr Rahman could see them. The memory clinic notes were there. The GP's latest observations were integrated.

Small things. Basic things. Made brilliant.

The hype hangover is real. But now you know how to navigate it.

Chapter 2
The Vocabulary Trap

Plain-Language Mental Models That Actually Work

Key message: You don't need to become a data scientist. You need enough vocabulary to ask intelligent questions, recognise evasive non-answers and make decisions based on understanding rather than faith in technical sophistication.

If You Read Nothing Else, Remember These Five Things

1. Jargon blocks scrutiny, and it's strategic, not accidental.

   When leaders can't distinguish "machine learning" from "automation", vendors hide limitations. When boards don't understand "external validation", they approve failures. The vocabulary trap works because accepting confusion feels easier than demanding clarity. The solution: Refuse to approve what you don't understand.

2. Most "AI" isn't.

   Only 10 – 15% of health care solutions marketed as "artificial intelligence" actually use machine learning. The rest is rules-based automation from the 1990s wearing new labels. Rules don't learn or adapt; they do exactly what they're programmed to do. Marketing them as "AI" creates expectations they'll never meet. Ask vendors, "Is this machine learning or rules-based?" If they can't answer clearly, walk away.

3. You need useful frameworks, not technical definitions.

   Think of AI as a pattern-spotter with PhD-level skills but zero judgement; it finds everything but understands nothing. A calculator that's faster but can't choose the problem to solve. A specialist consultant whose recommendations you evaluate critically, not accept blindly. Not perfect analogies. Useful ones that help you ask better questions.

4. Black boxes need clinical relevance, not perfect transparency.

   Deep learning can't always explain its reasoning. It can show which factors mattered but not why this particular combination triggered this particular alert. Demand outputs that connect to decisions: "Lactate rising, BP falling—consider sepsis" beats "Model confidence: 87%." If AI can't communicate clinically, it's not ready.

5. Four questions cut through any presentation.

   What patient outcome improves—not efficiency, actual benefit with evidence? How would clinicians use this in real practice—not demos, actual workflows? What happens when it fails—all systems fail, how does this one? Who monitors and maintains it—not during pilot, after scale? No clear answers? Don't proceed.

Opening

The Vendor Presentation

Two weeks after the board meeting, Samantha sits in another conference room. This time, she's ready to ask questions.

Twenty minutes into the vendor presentation, she knows how this ends.

The salesperson: "Our deep learning algorithms leverage transformer architectures for multimodal clinical inference..."

The chief medical officer (CMO) shifts. Glances at the chief nursing officer (CNO). Neither wants to admit confusion. The chief operating officer (COO) nods—he scheduled this meeting; can't look ignorant. The IT director checks email.

Samantha thinks about Dr Rahman, her mother's cardiologist. Last week he admitted the hospital's "AI-powered ECG system" baffles him. "It flags anomalies I'm supposed to review. Doesn't tell me what kind or why it matters. I click through most of them—no time investigating alerts I don't trust." The vendor continues, "The ensemble model combines gradient boosted decision trees with deep neural networks..."

The CMO interrupts. "Can you explain how this helps our doctors care for patients?"

Brief pause. Professional smile. "The platform uses advanced AI to improve decision-making through predictive analytics that leverage machine learning to identify patterns human clinicians might miss."

Not an answer. Jargon rearranged.

The CMO tries again. "What would a doctor actually do differently?"

Another pause. "They'd have access to insights generated by our proprietary algorithms, informing judgement with data-driven recommendations."

Still nothing concrete.

Samantha realises what she's watching. The jargon isn't accidental; it's defence. A way to prevent specific questions from exposing whether the vendor understands how their system works in real practice.

She considers asking, "Can you show exactly what appears on screen when a nurse is with a deteriorating patient at 3am?"

Decides against it. Not her meeting. The decision-makers should ask.

They don't.

Thirty minutes later: polite thanks, scheduled follow-up. The vendor leaves, confident.

As the room empties, the CNO to the CMO: "Didn't understand half of that, but it sounded impressive."

The CMO laughs uncomfortably. "Neither did I. But everyone else seems to think we need AI."

The jargon worked. Nobody asked what patient outcome would improve. Nobody asked about workflow integration. Nobody asked what happens when it fails.

They're about to approve something they don't understand.

Field Lesson 1: What "AI" Actually Means

The Uncomfortable Reality

Start with truth: Most systems marketed as "AI" in health care aren't artificial intelligence.

A 2024 Nature study analysing over 1,000 FDA-authorised AI medical devices found the agency uses "notably broad" definitions; some approved products use methods from the 1960s. Only 46% provide published performance data. The problem extends beyond health care. By 2024, the Securities and Exchange Commission (SEC) had started enforcing against "AI washing", with March penalties totalling $400,000 across two firms—Delphia and Global Predictions—making false AI claims.[4] Real machine learning—systems improving from experience without being explicitly reprogrammed—represents only 10 – 15% of health care solutions marketed as "AI." The rest is rules-based automation. If blood pressure is greater than 140 and age is greater than 65, then flag for hypertension. That's an algorithm. It might be sophisticated. But it's not AI. It doesn't learn. Doesn't adapt. Does exactly what it's programmed to do, nothing more.

Why This Matters

When health care leaders hear "AI-powered", they expect systems that learn and improve. Rules-based systems don't. They're deterministic—same inputs, same outputs, forever. This isn't inherently bad. Rules-based systems work well for many applications. But calling them "AI" creates expectation gaps that guarantee disappointment.

A hospital deployed "AI-powered bed management" expecting optimisation based on changing patient mix, seasonal patterns and practice evolution. The reality: preset rules. If discharge criteria are met, services are arranged and transport is confirmed, then flag as ready for discharge. No learning. No adaptation. Six months later, patient demographics shifted; there were more complex elderly patients with longer stays. The rules didn't adjust. Performance degraded. Leaders were confused: "Isn't AI supposed to improve?" If they'd known it was rules-based, they could have planned for regular rule updates. Expectations would have matched reality.

The Essential Distinctions

Understanding the spectrum matters more than memorising definitions, but leaders need enough clarity to ask the right questions.

Automation is technology performing tasks without human intervention: medication dispensing, appointment reminders, dosing calculators. It follows pre-programmed rules with zero learning.

Analytics uses statistical methods to find patterns: analysing readmission rates, identifying seasonal emergency department (ED) surges. It requires human interpretation and makes no autonomous decisions.

Machine learning trains algorithms on historical data to recognise patterns and predict outcomes. A sepsis prediction model learns which patients develop sepsis by studying thousands of cases, then predicts risk for new patients. It genuinely learns, but narrowly; sepsis prediction can't predict anything else.

Deep learning uses neural networks with many layers, excellent at complex patterns in large datasets like images, language and monitoring data. It's the least interpretable: It detects patterns humans miss but often can't explain why they matter. Generative AI is fundamentally different from all of these. Traditional AI classifies or predicts. Generative AI creates new content—drafting notes from conversation, suggesting treatments, answering questions. It's the most powerful and the least validated in health care.

Follow the practical test for leaders:

1. If it follows preset rules, it's automation, not AI. If it analyses historical data, it's analytics, not AI.
2. If it learns from data, it's machine learning—narrow AI.
3. If it creates new content, it's generative AI—the newest and least validated.

If the vendor just says "AI," ask, "Which type?" Their answer tells you more than the rest of their presentation.

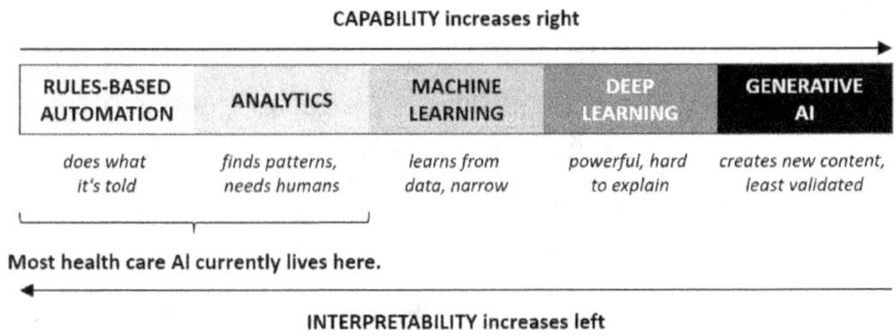

Figure 4. Most health care AI sits at the rules-based and analytics end. Capability increases right; interpretability increases left. Ask vendors which type before accepting the pitch.

Spotting the Jargon Trap

Certain phrases should trigger immediate scepticism. "Our proprietary algorithm leverages advanced machine learning" is dangerous because "proprietary" blocks scrutiny, "advanced" is meaningless and "leverages" says nothing about what it actually does. The counter-question: "Can you show me exactly what appears on screen when a clinician uses this system?"

"The platform provides intelligent insights through predictive analytics" sounds technical but communicates zero substance. What insights? What predictions? Based on what? Ask for a specific example: patient presentation, what the system outputs, what the clinician does differently.

"Our neural networks achieve 94% accuracy in clinical trials" matters because accuracy in controlled trials often crashes in real practice, and it doesn't specify the task or population. Ask what the accuracy was when deployed in real clinical settings with diverse patient populations.

"The system integrates seamlessly with existing workflows" is a reliable warning sign. Nothing integrates seamlessly. If they say it does, they haven't actually tested it. Ask them to walk through a workflow from clinician login to completed task, step by step. "This uses explainable AI, so clinicians can trust the recommendations" has become marketing shorthand. Real explainability requires showing which features mattered and connecting them to clinical reasoning. Ask to see an example of the explanation a clinician would actually receive.

There's a pattern to remember. When vendors use three layers of jargon to avoid one concrete example, they're hiding something—usually that the system doesn't work as promised or that they don't understand how it works in practice.

The Language Framework Problem

The same system gets described four different ways depending on who's talking. Regulatory teams call it "Software as Medical Device, Class II, Computer-Aided Detection for radiographic imaging". Data scientists describe "a convolutional neural network with attention mechanism, trained on 50,000 labelled X-rays." The vendor markets "an AI-powered imaging platform delivering intelligent insights for faster diagnosis". The radiologist using it daily says, "Software flagging suspicious areas for me to review." Each description is accurate. Each emphasises different aspects. When procurement, regulatory, technical and clinical teams aren't speaking compatible languages, they make incompatible decisions.

The solution isn't forcing identical vocabulary; different roles genuinely need different frames. The solution is translation. Someone in the organisation must ensure regulatory requirements, technical capabilities, vendor promises and clinical needs all describe the same system coherently. Without that translation function, decisions get made in silos and nobody notices they're talking about different things until the implementation fails.

Field Lesson 2: Mental Models That Work

You don't need to understand neural networks. You need mental models that connect technical capability to clinical reality.

The Brilliant Student with Zero Judgement

Think of machine learning as a brilliant medical student who's seen millions of cases but has no clinical judgement. Never sleeps. Never tires. Instantly recalls every case. Spots statistical patterns that would take humans years to notice. But has zero understanding of why patterns matter, what to do about them or how to handle cases that don't fit the pattern.

A machine learning system trained on 500,000 chest X-rays learns that particular combinations of opacity, location and borders appear in 73% of lung cancers and only 2% of benign cases. Flags this combination every time. Brilliant pattern recognition. But it doesn't understand anatomy. Show it an X-ray with a nodule in an anatomically impossible location and it might still flag it because the pattern matches. Show it a patient who had that lung removed and it might flag a "concerning nodule" in the missing lung. It finds the pattern. It can't understand the impossible context. This happened at a London teaching hospital in 2023. Their lung nodule detection system flagged "suspicious findings" in post-pneumonectomy patients, alerting radiologists to "concerning masses" in lungs that had been surgically removed years earlier. The AI found the pattern. It just couldn't understand the context.

The clinical implication is straightforward: Use machine learning for tireless pattern recognition, but don't expect clinical reasoning. Let it find things you should examine. You decide what the findings mean and what action to take.

The Calculator for Diagnosis

Calculators are faster, more consistent and make fewer errors than humans. Extremely useful. But you need to know what to calculate, whether the answer makes sense and what to do with the result. A calculator showing cardiac output as negative 47 litres per minute hasn't malfunctioned. Someone entered wrong inputs or asked the wrong question. The calculator calculated. The error was in the human-calculator interaction.

AI works identically. It performs tasks faster and more consistently but doesn't understand the problem you're solving. Doesn't know whether inputs make sense. Can't judge whether outputs are reasonable. Edinburgh's stroke prevention programme learnt this the hard way. Their AI calculated perfect CHA_2DS_2-VASc scores (Atrial Fibrillation Stroke Risk) from EMR data. Six months in, an audit revealed 23% had incomplete medication histories—patients taking anticoagulants that weren't recorded. The AI calculated scores assuming no anticoagulation, recommending treatments patients were already receiving. The maths was perfect. The inputs were garbage.

The clinical implication: AI can calculate, classify and predict faster than humans. It cannot understand context, recognise when standard approaches don't apply or know what to do with results. Those remain human responsibilities.

The Specialist Consultant

"AI as co-pilot" has become popular shorthand. It works well for some applications and misleads for others.

Where it works: ambient documentation, where AI transcribes and structures conversation while the clinician focuses on the patient. Clear division of labour. The clinician reviews and finalises. Accountability is clear. Genuine co-piloting. Kaiser Permanente's ambient documentation saved 15,791 hours—approximately seven working years—across over 2.5 million encounters. Clinicians report that for the first time in years, they can look at their patient instead of typing. Where it misleads: complex treatment decisions, where AI suggests treatments and the question becomes who's actually piloting. If the clinician almost always accepts, who's making the decision? If they frequently override, what value is the AI adding? In high-stakes emergencies, clinicians may defer without adequate evaluation. That's not co-piloting; it's automation bias, where the human becomes co-pilot to the AI.

The better framing is AI as specialist consultant. When a generalist consults a specialist, they don't blindly accept recommendations. They understand the reasoning, consider the whole-patient context and make the final decision. Sometimes they agree. Sometimes they don't. This consultant framing clarifies that recommendations require critical evaluation, not automatic acceptance. Accountability remains with the treating clinician, matching medical-legal reality. Melbourne's Royal Hospital learnt this through painful experience. They deployed an AI sepsis prediction system framed as a "co-pilot". Within three months, nursing staff reported feeling pressured to escalate every AI alert—"The system is the expert. Who am I to question it?" False positive rates climbed to 67%". Alert fatigue set in. Staff started ignoring alerts entirely. The hospital reframed it as a "specialist consultant" and retrained staff: "This is like calling infectious diseases or critical care for input. They give recommendations. You integrate with everything else you know about the patient. You make the call." Escalation decisions improved. Nurses felt empowered to use clinical judgement. The technology didn't change. The framing did.

Field Lesson 3: The Black Box Reality

What We Can and Cannot Explain

The black box problem is real but widely misunderstood. It's not binary—transparent versus opaque. It's a spectrum of interpretability challenges, and the practical question isn't whether we can explain everything but whether we can explain enough.

What we can explain: feature importance—which variables mattered most, whether age, blood pressure or laboratory results. Modern AI ranks the relative importance of inputs. Similar cases—for this prediction, here are patients from the training data with similar profiles and their outcomes. This provides context even without explaining exact reasoning. Confidence levels—how certain is the system? 95% versus 60%? Uncertainty quantification is genuinely valuable. Decision boundaries—at what threshold does the AI change its recommendation? If blood pressure were 10 points lower, would the recommendation change? These are testable.

What we often cannot explain: precise reasoning paths in deep learning with millions of parameters across dozens of layers. There's no simple explanation for why this particular input combination produced that particular output. The model learnt patterns that are mathematically describable but not intuitively understandable. Complex interaction effects how features interact with each other. Age might affect outcomes differently depending on blood pressure, which is affected differently depending on medications, which interacts with genetic factors. AI captures these complex interactions, but explaining them in plain language is often impossible.

Explainability Versus Interpretability

These are different things, and the distinction matters.

Explainability provides post-hoc rationalisation. After the AI decides, we analyse which features influenced the decision, how it compares to similar cases and what would change the outcome. We're describing what the AI did, not understanding why.

Interpretability means understanding the model's actual decision process. Simple models—decision trees, linear regression—are interpretable. Complex deep learning often isn't.

Health care doesn't necessarily need perfect interpretability. It needs clinical relevance.

What Clinicians Actually Need

Compare outputs. "Model detected pattern score 0.87 based on weighted combination of 47 variables" tells a clinician nothing actionable. "Deterioration risk increased over the past six hours. Key changes: lactate rising—3.2, was 1.8. BP falling—systolic 92, was 118. Heart rate increasing—118, was 88. Consider sepsis workup"—that connects to clinical decision-making. "Neural network confidence: 94%" is meaningless in isolation. "This pattern appears in 94% of patients who later developed complications. However, 12% with this pattern did not deteriorate; clinical judgement recommended" respects the clinician's role. "Algorithm classified this X-ray as abnormal" is incomplete. "Opacity detected right lower lobe consistent with pneumonia. However, it could also represent atelectasis or prior scarring. Recommend clinical correlation and comparison with previous imaging" integrates with how clinicians actually think. The difference is clinical context. AI that doesn't just report what it found but provides information connecting to clinical decision-making. Some organisations achieve this by building translation layers—software that takes AI outputs and reformats them for clinical relevance. Others involve clinicians in designing exactly what information the AI should surface and how. The best solutions combine both. The black box becomes less of a barrier when AI communicates like a clinician instead of a mathematician.

Field Lesson 4: Building Shared Language

Twelve Terms That Matter

You don't need to become a data scientist. You need enough vocabulary to ask intelligent questions and recognise non-answers. Twelve terms provide the foundation:

1. "Algorithm" is a rule set for solving a problem.

   It can be simple;—if blood pressure is greater than 140, flag hypertension—or complex, drawing on learnt patterns from millions of patients. Algorithm is recipe, not magic. When vendors say "our algorithm", ask, "What problem does it solve and how?"

2. "Training data" is the historical examples AI learns from.

   If trained only on academic centre data, it may not work in community hospitals. If trained only on one demographic, it may perform poorly for others. AI can't learn what it hasn't seen. Ask, "What data was this trained on? Is it similar to our population?"

3. "Validation" tests whether AI works.

   Internal validation uses the same environment where it was developed. External validation tests completely different settings—different hospitals, populations, workflows. External is the gold standard and is surprisingly rare. Always ask, "Has this been externally validated in settings like ours?"

4. "Bias" means systematic errors favouring some groups over others.

   If trained mainly on men's data, it may perform worse for women. If trained in well-resourced hospitals, it may fail in under-resourced ones. Bias isn't a fixable bug; it's baked into the data and requires constant vigilance. Ask. "What populations was this validated on? How does performance vary across demographics?"

5. "Model drift" is performance degrading over time because the patterns the system learnt no longer match current reality.

   Clinical practices evolve. Patient populations shift. Last year's accurate algorithm may fail this year. Drift requires ongoing monitoring and periodic retraining. Ask, "Who monitors for drift and how often is retraining planned?"

6. "False positive" is when the AI says something's wrong when it isn't.

   Too many create alert fatigue; clinicians learn to ignore alerts and miss the real ones. Ask, "What's the false positive rate in real-world use?"

7. "False negative" is when the AI misses something actually wrong.

   These are invisible failures unless specifically measured. Ask, "What's the false negative rate and how was it measured?"

8. "Confidence score" is the AI's certainty estimate.

   Ninety-five per cent confidence sounds impressive but means it is wrong 5% of the time. For rare conditions, even high confidence can mean frequent errors. Confidence isn't correctness; it's the AI's estimate based on training data and may not match your population. Ask, "How was confidence calibrated for our population?"

9. "Feature" is a measurable characteristic used for prediction.

   Age is a feature. Blood pressure is a feature. Laboratory values are features. Understanding which features matter helps you know which data quality issues will break the system. Ask, "Which features does this use and why?"

10. "Inference" is what the AI does in real time—taking new data and producing predictions.

    Training is learning from historical data. Inference is applying those learnt patterns to new patients. Fast inference matters when you need real-time recommendations. Ask, "How fast is inference and where does computation happen?"

11. "Ground truth" is the "correct answer" used to train and validate AI.

    For imaging, ground truth might be expert consensus or biopsy results. But ground truth is often imperfect—experts disagree, tests have errors. AI trained on imperfect ground truth learns imperfect patterns. Ask, "What was the ground truth and how reliable is it?"

12. "Generalisation" describes how well AI performs on new, unseen data.

    A system might achieve 99% accuracy on training data but only 75% on new patients; it memorised training-specific patterns rather than learning generalisable ones. External validation tests generalisation. Ask, "How well did this generalise to populations different from training?"

These 12 terms won't make you a technical expert. They'll make you a more effective questioner, and in health care AI, that matters more.

Framework Close: From Confusion to Clarity

The presentation ends. Executives file out. Samantha returns to her desk and opens her laptop.

She drafts an email to the medical director:

Subject: Questions about the AI vendor proposal.

Before proceeding, I think we should ask the vendor to clarify four things:

1. What specific patient outcome will improve if we deploy this—not efficiency metrics, actual patient benefit?
2. How exactly would a clinician use this in real workflow, not ideal demo conditions?
3. What happens when the system is wrong, and how would clinicians know?
4. Who owns ongoing monitoring and maintenance after the implementation team moves to the next project?

If they can't answer these clearly, I'm not confident we understand what we're buying.

She hesitates. Not her lane. She's supposed to take notes, not question experts.

But she thinks about Dr Rahman, clicking through AI alerts he doesn't trust. The jargon-heavy presentation where nobody asked hard questions. Systems she's watched fail because leaders approved complexity they didn't understand.

She sends the email.

The medical director replies within an hour:

"Thank you. Exactly right. I'll send these questions to the vendor now and tell them we need answers before the next meeting. If they can't explain their system clearly, we don't need it."

Samantha feels something shift. The vocabulary trap can be escaped. But only if someone is willing to say, "I don't understand this, and I need you to explain it differently."

That permission to not understand—to demand clarity instead of accepting confusion—might be the most important thing she's learnt.

Remember the Five Things

These aren't five separate lessons. They're a connected system, and the connection matters.

1. Jargon blocks scrutiny.

   When executives can't distinguish machine learning from automation, vendors hide limitations behind technical sophistication. They refuse to approve what you don't understand. If a vendor can't explain their system in language your clinical staff would use, it's not ready.

2. Most "AI" isn't.

   Only 10 – 15% of health care solutions marketed as AI actually use machine learning. Ask vendors directly, "Is this machine learning or rules-based?" If they can't answer clearly, walk away. The question saves millions.

3. The Permanente Medical Group.

   The brilliant student, the calculator, the specialist consultant—these framings connect AI capability to clinical reality. Use them in board discussions. They change the conversation from "How impressive is this?" to "How would we actually use this?"

4. Demand clinical relevance from black boxes.

   Deep learning can't always explain its reasoning, but it can show which factors mattered and connect outputs to clinical decisions. "Lactate rising, BP falling—consider sepsis" is what clinicians need. If AI can't communicate clinically, it's not ready.

5. Ask the four questions before every decision.

   What patient outcome improves? How would clinicians use this in real practice? What happens when it fails? Who monitors and maintains it after scale? No clear answers? Don't proceed.

The next chapter addresses the uncomfortable truth that vocabulary clarity reveals: Most health care systems aren't ready for AI. Not because their data quality is poor, though often it is. But because the infrastructure connecting their fragments doesn't exist. Connection before intelligence isn't just a principle. It's the difference between pilots that impress and systems that transform.

Chapter 3
The Uncomfortable Truth

What Leaders Need to See Before They Sign

Key message: Before building, leaders need to see what business cases rarely show them—the real cost of integration, the evidence gaps behind confident projections and the organisational readiness that determines whether technology reaches patients. Seeing clearly isn't pessimism. It's the foundation for building wisely. The evidence we need is still being built; that's not a reason to wait but a reason to move forward honestly, learning as we go.

If You Read Nothing Else, Remember These Five Things

1. Most health care AI shows no calculable ROI.

   Only 5% of implementations demonstrate clear financial returns. Not because AI lacks value—because measuring that value against implementation costs, ongoing maintenance and opportunity costs reveals complexity vendors prefer avoiding. This isn't failure. It's honest assessment revealing why Chapter 1's validation questions matter.

2. The integration iceberg sinks most pilots.

   Between 80 and 92% of pilots fail to scale, primarily because nobody budgeted for the EMR/EHR integration work that determines success. Integration requires three to five times initial software costs—custom APIs, data transformation, workflow redesign, ongoing maintenance. Vendors quote licensing. Reality requires platform building.

3. The talent gap is widening, not closing.

   Health care needs thousands of clinical informaticists and AI-literate clinicians. Fewer than 20% of organisations have systematic training programmes or defined career paths. Organisations building talent systematically sustain transformation. The best consulting relationships build organisational muscle, not reliance. If your consulting engagement doesn't have a defined exit point and a capability transfer plan, you're buying a service, not building a future.

4. AI deployment without equity analysis amplifies existing disparities.

   Fewer than 15% of implementations include systematic bias testing across demographic groups. Algorithms trained predominantly on majority populations perform poorly for minorities, yet most organisations deploy without demographic validation. Remember the dermatology AI from

Chapter 1: internal accuracy of 88 – 94% collapsed to 56 – 67% on diverse patients.

5. Change management determines outcomes more than technology.

   Implementations without clinical champion networks, workflow integration plans and ongoing governance fail even when the AI works perfectly. Technology is the easy part. The human dimension determines whether investments deliver value.

Opening

The Governance Meeting

Samantha finds herself in a governance committee meeting reviewing quarterly AI pilot performance. Seven active implementations on the agenda. She spent the previous evening reading performance reports and financial summaries, noting what was measured and, more importantly, what wasn't.

The IT director presents first. Adoption rates climbing. User satisfaction positive. No major technical incidents. Finance confirms all projects tracking to budget. The CMO reports clinical staff are "generally supportive". Slides advance. Heads nod.

Samantha raises her hand. "Can someone explain the actual patient outcomes for these implementations? Not adoption metrics, clinical outcomes. Did readmissions decrease? Did wait times improve?" The IT director scans his presentation for data that isn't there. The CMO acknowledges outcome measurement wasn't included in the initial deployment plans. The quality director mentions they've been "meaning to look at that".

"So we've spent £4.7 million implementing seven AI tools, and we can't say whether any of them improved patient care?"

The CEO thanks Samantha for the challenge and suggests the programme office review how outcome metrics might be incorporated going forward. The meeting moves on. Samantha writes in her notebook: "Outcome metrics—follow up". She knows what "review going forward" means in NHS governance.

Walking to her office afterwards, a voice behind her: "Good question in there."

She turns. Ravi Chandrasekaran, the external advisor the board brought in three months ago to review their AI portfolio. His background preceded him: 15 years implementing health care technology across the Gulf, Southeast Asia and the UK. Most recently he'd led digital health strategy for a large hospital group in Abu Dhabi, one of the few systems that had actually scaled AI beyond pilots. The trust hired him because the board wanted an honest assessment of whether their investments were delivering. From what she'd heard, they weren't entirely sure they wanted the answer. "Fat lot of good it did," she says. "You know why nobody answered it properly? Because answering it means admitting that three or four of those implementations should probably be paused. Nobody wants to say we spent £4.7 million on tools we can't prove are helping patients. It's easier to measure adoption and call it progress."

"So what do we do?"

"Keep asking. Every meeting. Make it boring. Make it the thing people expect so they start preparing the answer before they walk in." He pauses. "The organisations that get this right don't have a breakthrough moment. They just stop accepting comfortable metrics as evidence of impact."

She thinks about Margaret. Three hospital systems. Four patient portals. None of them talking to each other. How many AI tools have touched her mother's care? How many made things better versus just different?

Nobody knows. Not really.

Field Lesson 1: The Evidence Gap

The ROI Questions Without Answers

Ask vendors for ROI evidence and watch presentations pivot quickly from financial returns to "strategic value" and "competitive positioning". The uncomfortable truth is that only 5% of health care AI implementations can demonstrate calculable financial returns. Not because AI lacks value but because measuring that value against implementation costs, ongoing maintenance and opportunity costs reveals complexity that vendors prefer avoiding.

A large hospital group in the Gulf implemented an AI scheduling system promising 15% efficiency gains in outpatient clinics. Eighteen months later, their finance team couldn't isolate any measurable improvement in throughput, revenue or patient satisfaction scores. The AI worked; appointments were scheduled. But did it deliver value exceeding its $3.2 million implementation cost plus $600,000 annual licensing? Nobody could say definitively.

This isn't failure. It's an honest assessment. The system improved workflow for some specialties while creating bottlenecks for others. Staff needed six months adapting to new processes, during which productivity actually declined. Integration required custom development nobody budgeted for—another $1.1 million. When you account for real costs against claimed benefits, ROI becomes muddy. The problem isn't the technology. It's the methodology. Traditional business cases assume well-defined independent variables—change X, measure Y. But health care AI involves what economists call entanglement; everything affects everything else. Vendor business cases isolate benefits while socialising costs. They credit the AI with any efficiency gain while attributing costs elsewhere—integration to IT budgets, training to HR, change management to operations. This accounting sleight of hand makes almost any investment appear justified.

Outcomes Versus Efficiency: The Validation Challenge

Vendor demonstrations often showcase impressive efficiency metrics: reduced documentation time, faster triage, fewer clicks per order. But health care leaders need outcomes evidence: reduced readmissions, improved survival rates, better patient experience, lower total cost of care. These metrics require years to accumulate and rigorous study designs to validate. Most vendors lack them.

In 2022, Stanford and Memorial Sloan Kettering Cancer Centre researchers tested three commercially available dermatology AI algorithms—tools already approved by European regulators and marketed to clinicians—on a diverse clinical dataset with pathologically confirmed diagnoses. The algorithms claimed impressive accuracy. Internal validation showed AUC scores of 0.88 – 0.94. For context, AUC measures how well an algorithm distinguishes between conditions;1.0 is perfect and 0.5 is random chance. Scores above 0.85 typically appear in vendor presentations as evidence of clinical-grade performance.

External validation told a different story. When tested on the Diverse Dermatology Images dataset—photographs reflecting actual patient diversity—performance dropped dramatically. AUC scores fell to 0.56 – 0.67, a 27 – 36% decline from reported performance, approaching random chance for some patient groups. More concerning was what the study revealed about equity.[5] DeepDerm performed at essentially random chance on dark skin—

AUC 0.50—while achieving 0.61 on light skin. For detecting malignancy, the algorithm showed 69% sensitivity on light skin versus just 23% on dark skin. The good news is when the algorithms were fine-tuned on diverse data, performance gaps closed significantly. The problem was solvable but only once it was visible.

The Replication Crisis and Publication Bias

Academic medicine faces a replication crisis that directly affects AI validation. Algorithms performing impressively in development environments often struggle in real-world deployment. Research datasets are carefully curated: high-quality images, expert-confirmed diagnoses, controlled conditions. Clinical data is messy: variable image quality, uncertain diagnoses, complex patient populations that don't match training data demographics.

The problem compounds because negative results rarely get published. Failed pilots disappear quietly. Successful deployments generate case studies and conference presentations. This publication bias creates distorted perceptions; leaders see success stories while failures remain invisible, leading to unrealistic expectations.

The path forward: Frame this as "structured experimentation with appropriate oversight". Not every AI deployment will succeed. Not every vendor claim will materialise. The question isn't whether failures will occur but whether organisations learn from them systematically. Chapter 1's validation framework, demanding external validation in settings like yours, becomes essential here. Build the muscle for honest assessment before investing at scale.

Field Lesson 2: The Integration Iceberg

Why Brilliant AI Dies in Integration

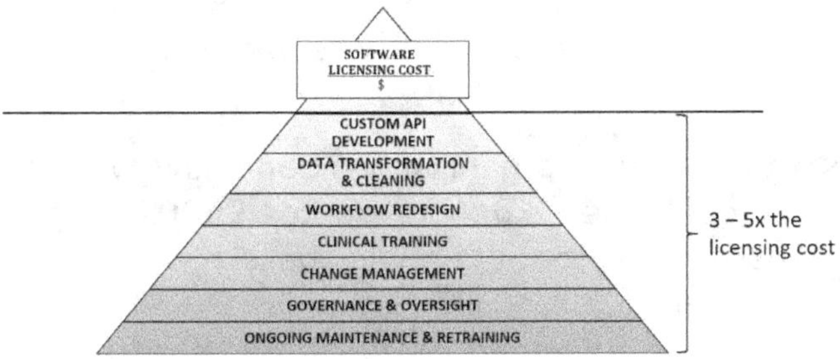

Figure 5. Software licensing is the visible tip. The hidden mass—API development, data cleaning, workflow redesign, training, change management, governance—runs 3 to 5 times the licensing cost.

Health care AI's biggest failure point isn't algorithm performance; it's integration. Eighty to 92% of pilots fail to scale to production. The primary cause: inadequate integration planning and resourcing. Pilots succeed technically but die attempting to work within the systems clinicians actually use every day.

The Microsoft-Nuance story from Chapter 1 illustrates what even success requires. Microsoft spent $19.7 billion acquiring Nuance. They had deep health care expertise and frontier AI capability and achieved Epic compatibility in under six months. By any measure, this is health care AI done right. Yet even they discovered that licensing the software was the easy part. Making it work meant redesigning clinical workflows, training thousands of clinicians, mapping the technology to how each hospital actually operates and maintaining all of it as systems update. Microsoft budgeted for that complexity. That's why the acquisition made sense at $19.7 billion; they knew the integration work was where the real cost lived.

Most health care organisations don't have Microsoft's resources. When a vendor quotes £500,000 annual licensing, finance approves based on efficiency projections. Then IT receives the integration requirements and estimates 18 months of development work and three full-time staff—another £2.2 million. Suddenly, £500,000 becomes £2.7 million. And that's before training, workflow redesign and ongoing maintenance. The lesson isn't that Microsoft overspent. It's that typical vendor evaluations dramatically underestimate what integration actually costs.

The Platform Question Nobody Asks

Most health care organisations lack AI-ready infrastructure. Implementing point solutions one by one creates technical debt that compounds over time. Each tool requires custom integration. Each generates proprietary data formats. Each demands separate maintenance workflows. After deploying five AI tools, organisations discover they're maintaining five custom integration pipelines. Forward-thinking organisations invest in platform capabilities before deploying multiple AI solutions. They build unified data models allowing different tools to share standardised inputs. They develop API frameworks enabling plug-and-play integration. They establish governance structures providing consistent oversight. Organisations that build platforms first deploy subsequent AI tools faster and at 60 – 70% lower cost.

But platform thinking carries its own risks. Three-year data lake projects that never reach completion. Infrastructure investments that become outdated before delivering value. The answer isn't choosing between platforms and point solutions; it's sequencing correctly. Start with one critical problem. Solve it in six to eight weeks using existing infrastructure. Then let each solution become a building block for the platform rather than waiting for perfect infrastructure before solving any problems. Chapter 4 explores this in detail.

Critical Systems Risk and the Safety Imperative

Health care IT operates in a zero-error-tolerance environment. Systems going down means patients at risk. Integration work involving critical clinical systems requires extensive testing, rollback planning and phased deployment. Vendors accustomed to commercial software deployment timelines underestimate health care's necessary caution.

A 600-bed hospital in the Gulf Cooperation Council (GCC) planned a six-month deployment for an AI-powered medication reconciliation system. Eighteen months later, they were still in testing. Not because the AI failed; it worked perfectly in isolated testing environments. But integration revealed edge cases nobody anticipated: complex medication regimens misinterpreted, drug databases using different naming conventions, alerts firing in inappropriate contexts.

The path forward: budget three to five times software costs for integration work. Treat EMRs as evolving partners, not barriers; Epic, Cerner and Oracle are all building AI capabilities themselves. Learn from their experience implementing at scale. The integration iceberg kills pilots, but organisations that plan for it realistically turn it into competitive advantage.

Field Lesson 3: Talent, Equity and Liability

The Talent Gap Nobody's Solving

Health care organisations need two talent categories for successful AI deployment: clinical informaticists who bridge clinical practice and technical implementation and AI-literate clinicians who can evaluate tools, lead adoption and provide ongoing governance. Most organisations have neither in sufficient numbers.

A typical large hospital system might employ one or two clinical informaticists supporting hundreds of clinicians. These individuals become bottlenecks as AI tools proliferate. As one informaticist described, "I'm supporting seven active AI implementations, evaluating three proposals and helping troubleshoot two systems showing performance drift, meaning their accuracy is degrading over time as patient populations and clinical practices change. I'm supposed to be full-time on each of these."

The solution requires systematically developing internal capabilities: formal training programmes, career pathways that reward clinical informatics expertise and protected time for skill development. Few organisations have built these elements. External consultants can provide temporary support but can't replace organisational competence.

Equity Implications Being Ignored

AI trained predominantly on data from majority populations can perform poorly for minority groups, yet systematic bias testing remains rare. A Stanford study analysing FDA-approved AI medical devices found that fewer than 15% reported performance metrics stratified by race or ethnicity.[6]

This matters clinically. A pulse oximetry algorithm trained primarily on light-skinned patients showed reduced accuracy for patients with darker skin tones, potentially leading to delayed recognition of hypoxemia. Dermatology AI trained on images from practices where patients are disproportionately white struggles to identify skin conditions in darker skin. Cardiac risk prediction algorithms trained on data lacking adequate minority representation may underestimate risk in those populations.

Addressing equity concerns requires demanding demographic stratification in vendor validation studies, conducting local bias testing before deployment, monitoring performance disparities after implementation and refusing to deploy tools showing clinically significant performance gaps. These requirements add cost. But deploying AI that performs unequally across populations violates fundamental health care obligations.

The Liability Vacuum and Risk Allocation

When AI contributes to patient harm, who bears liability? This question lacks clear answers. Vendor contracts typically limit liability to software licensing costs. Health care organisations bear patient care responsibility. But if an AI tool's erroneous output leads a clinician to make a harmful decision, the liability becomes murky.

Consider this scenario: An AI prediction tool generates an alert that a patient has low risk for deterioration. The clinician, trusting the system, delays ordering additional tests. The patient deteriorates rapidly and suffers significant harm. Investigation reveals the AI missed warning signs because the patient's presentation was unusual, not technically a failure since the algorithm performed within specifications but clinically a disaster.

There's no black-and-white answer here. The skill is assembling the right combination of safeguards for your context. A practical liability toolkit has several components:

- deploy in phases, with governance checkpoints before each stage expands;
- define the risk thresholds where a human must be in the loop and don't compromise on them;
- document every decision in vendor evaluation and deployment so due diligence is visible, not assumed;

- structure insurance and indemnification to cover AI-augmented care specifically. Participate in regulatory sandboxes where they exist and
- build kill-switch protocols before you need them. Deciding how to pause an underperforming system during a crisis is too late.

The path forward: frame this as "structured experimentation with appropriate oversight". This framing honours legitimate legal concerns while enabling organisations to learn and improve. Few organisations have invested in building these governance elements, but those that do create a sustainable advantage.

Field Lesson 4: Change Management Determines Success

Technology Is the Easy Part

The most common implementation failure mode: perfect technology, failed adoption. AI tools work exactly as designed, yet clinicians don't use them. A radiology department deploys an AI reading assistant that accurately flags abnormal findings. Six months later, usage analytics show 40% of radiologists rarely activate it. When asked why, the response is, "It slows me down more than it helps." Change management separates successful deployments from expensive disappointments. Successful implementations share common patterns: clinical champions leading adoption within departments, workflow analysis preceding deployment, iterative rollout allowing refinement, ongoing feedback mechanisms letting users shape how the tool evolves and protected time for learning without compromising patient care. These change management elements—training programmes, protected time, champion compensation— cost money. Then implementations stumble because nobody planned for the human dimension of technological change.

The Governance Vacuum

Who decides when an AI tool isn't performing adequately? Who monitors for performance drift over time? Who has the authority to pause or retire underperforming systems? These governance questions lack clear answers in most organisations.

A health system deployed a readmissions prediction model in 2024. Initially, it performed well. Twelve months after deployment, a quality improvement team noticed readmission rates weren't declining as projected. Investigation revealed the model had drifted; patient acuity had increased, discharge patterns had changed and social services availability had decreased. The model hadn't adapted. Nobody was watching. Effective AI governance requires clear accountability structures defining decision rights, performance monitoring systems tracking key metrics continuously, regular review processes evaluating tool value against costs, escalation procedures addressing performance concerns and sunset policies allowing graceful retirement of underperforming tools. Without active governance, deployed tools gradually lose relevance while consuming ongoing costs.

Alert Fatigue and the Maintenance Reality

Clinical decision support tools generate alerts. Too many alerts create fatigue; clinicians start dismissing warnings reflexively. A cardiac risk prediction system initially generated 12 helpful alerts daily across a 300-bed hospital. Six months later, the system was generating 47 alerts daily, many of them false positives. Clinical staff said, “The tool cried wolf too often. We stopped trusting it.”

Managing this requires baseline alert volume assessment before deployment, false positive rate monitoring after implementation, regular tuning to maintain the optimal sensitivity-specificity balance and user feedback mechanisms identifying alerts that clinicians find unhelpful. These maintenance activities represent ongoing work that nobody budgets for initially.

The path forward sounds simple but requires a fight most leaders aren’t expecting: getting change management funded as seriously as technology. Finance committees approve software licensing without hesitation. Ask for the same amount for training programmes, protected clinician time and governance staffing, and the conversation changes entirely. “Can’t we just absorb that into existing roles?” You can’t. The organisations that try end up with perfect technology nobody uses. The practical move is to include change management and governance as line items in the original business case, not as a follow-up request after the technology is approved. Bundle them so they can’t be stripped out during budget review. If the total cost—technology plus integration plus change management plus governance—doesn't survive scrutiny, the project wasn’t viable in the first place. Better to know that before you’ve spent the money. Plan for ongoing governance from day one. Build feedback loops that let clinicians shape how tools evolve. And remember the question from Chapter 1: “Who owns this when the champion leaves?” It applies here with full force. Technology without governance creates expensive disappointments.

Framework Close: Honest Questions Before Your Next AI Decision

Before approving any AI procurement or scaling decision, the leadership team should be able to answer five questions clearly. If they can’t, the organisation doesn’t have enough information to proceed.

1. What evidence would we need to see before scaling this investment, and does that evidence exist anywhere?

2. Have we budgeted three to five times software costs for integration, or are we pretending licensing is the total cost?
3. Is this vendor relationship creating joint value, or is one party extracting value without reciprocal investment?
4. Who will govern this system after deployment, and what authority do they have to pause or retire it?
5. What's our liability toolkit for this implementation, and have legal, clinical and technical leaders agreed on it?

Back to Samantha

Two weeks after the governance meeting, Samantha sits across from Ravi in the hospital café. She'd asked for this conversation, not as operations director meeting consultant but as someone trying to make sense of what she'd uncovered.

"The thing that bothers me," she says, "is that we spent £4.7 million and nobody can tell me whether patients are better off."

Ravi stirs his coffee. Doesn't rush to answer.

"I ran a digital health programme for a large hospital group in the Gulf. Well-funded, leadership committed. We deployed 11 AI tools in 18 months. I was proud of it—presented it at conferences, wrote it up, the whole thing." He sets down his spoon. "Then one of my team, younger than me, braver than me, asked your question. Not 'Are the tools working?' but 'Which patient outcomes changed because of them?' I knew things were better. I could feel it in the wards. But when she pushed me to separate what the AI had done from everything else we'd changed—new workflows, extra staff, better processes—I couldn't. Not cleanly. Eleven tools. Eighteen months. And the honest answer was, something's working, but we don't know exactly what."

"So what did you do?"

"Stopped deploying and started connecting. That was the shift. We'd been treating each tool as a standalone project—separate vendor, separate integration, separate governance. The AI worked fine. The systems couldn't see each other." He looks at her. "Sound familiar?"

Samantha almost laughs. Seventeen pilots at her trust. None connected.

"The problem was never the technology. It was that we had no platform underneath. No shared data layer. No common way for these tools to see the same patient. Every deployment started from scratch." He leans forward. "Your trust isn't failing because you chose the wrong tools. You're failing because each one exists in isolation. Connect them and they start compounding. Leave them disconnected and you'll keep measuring adoption and calling it progress."

Samantha thinks about Margaret. Last Tuesday, her mother's cardiologist increased a medication and the memory clinic didn't know. Not a technology problem. A connection problem.

"Where do we start?"

"One problem that matters enough to build the connections for. Not 11 tools. One problem, solved properly, and then you've got infrastructure that makes the next one easier." It's not the answer she wanted. She wanted a checklist, a roadmap. Instead she got a story about someone else's failure and a principle she'll have to figure out how to apply. But hearing Ravi—someone with 15 years and a track record she respected—admit he'd got it wrong makes her feel less alone in not having the answers.

That, she realises, is exactly what uncomfortable truths are for. Not to paralyse you. To show you where to look next.

Remember the Five Things

These aren't five separate problems. They're a connected system, and until you see the connections, you'll keep solving one while the others undermine you.

1. Honest ROI assessment matters more than optimistic projections.

Organisations measuring real costs and benefits make better decisions than those accepting vendor business cases uncritically. Fund implementations for strategic value with eyes open, not pretending certainty exists when it doesn't. Apply Chapter 1's four questions before every decision.

2. Integration planning determines success more than algorithm performance.

   Budget three to five times software costs for integration work. The integration iceberg kills 80 – 92% of pilots, but organisations that plan for it realistically turn constraint into advantage. Chapter 4 will show you how to build platforms that make integration progressively easier.

3. Building internal capabilities beats hiring consultants.

   Organisations developing clinical informatics talent and AI-literate clinical leaders sustain transformation beyond individual projects. External expertise supplements but can't replace organisational competence. Start building now; the talent gap is widening.

4. Equity analysis isn't optional; it's fundamental to health care's mission.

   Tools performing unequally across demographic groups harm patients and violate health care's core obligations. Demand demographic stratification in vendor studies. Test locally.

Monitor continuously. The dermatology AI validation failure showed the problem is solvable but only when visible.

5. Change management and governance cost more than technology and matter more.

   Organisations investing in clinician engagement, workflow integration and ongoing governance achieve adoption that organisations focusing purely on technical deployment never reach. The human dimension determines whether expensive pilots deliver lasting value. These uncomfortable truths create decision clarity. Once leaders see accurately—acknowledging evidence gaps, integration complexity, talent requirements, equity obligations and change management realities; they can build wisely.

Part II provides frameworks for that building. Chapter 4 introduces the operating system mindset—thinking differently about infrastructure, moving from service delivery to platform, delivering quarterly value rather than three-year promises. Chapter 5 explores ontologies: how AI learns to understand health care's complexity. Chapter 6 develops augmentation strategies balancing human and machine capabilities. Chapter 7 addresses workforce development supporting transformation. But building requires first seeing clearly. That's what these uncomfortable truths enable.

PART II: BUILDING WISELY

Chapter 4
The Operating System

Building the Platform that Makes Everything Else Possible

Key message: The shift isn't about more technology. It's about thinking differently—from service delivery to platform, from projects to operating system. Health care organisations spending years building perfect infrastructure watch their problems evolve and stakeholders change while they build. Meanwhile, organisations solving one critical problem in six to eight weeks, then expanding systematically, deliver quarterly value while building platforms from successful use cases. Brilliant basics, brilliantly executed.

If You Read Nothing Else, Remember These Five Things

1. Platform thinking beats project thinking, but platforms must grow from success, not precede it.

   Organisations solving one critical problem in six to eight weeks using existing infrastructure, then expanding systematically, outperform those spending three years building perfect data lakes. Your operating system should emerge from successful use cases that deliver immediate value alongside architectural planning that evolves with what you learn. Kaiser Permanente's multi-year IT modernisation worked because it integrated cloud solutions with immediate clinical value, saving $1.5 billion annually through genuine platform effects, not from infrastructure deployed hoping applications would follow.

2. Infrastructure before applications, but only if infrastructure enables timely value delivery.

   Estonia's X-Road shows the discipline required: seven years building secure data exchange infrastructure before launching the national electronic health record. That patience created foundations now processing 2.2 billion transactions yearly across 100% of residents' digital health records with 99% digital prescriptions. But even during those seven years, X-Road enabled incremental services. Infrastructure investment without quarterly visible value typically means you're building the wrong infrastructure.

3. Integration work determines success more than algorithm sophistication. Budget accordingly.

   NHS Fife's Morse (EPR) integration with the Orion Health portal eliminated duplicate appointment entries and gave clinicians complete patient views across community and acute systems. That integration work, not the

EPR software itself, created value. Integration costs will exceed technology costs by a factor for most implementations. Organisations treating integration as an afterthought repeat the 80 – 92% pilot failure rate from Chapter 3. Those planning for integration complexity from day one build platforms that make subsequent integrations progressively easier.

4. Data quality is necessary but not sufficient. Iterative improvement beats waiting for perfection.

   Nordic countries processing millions of health transactions daily show the reality: 20 – 30% structured data, 70 – 80% unstructured. Denmark's Sundhed.dk launched in 2003 and has continuously evolved for over two decades through systematic improvement cycles. Finland's Kanta platform represents 20 years of ecosystem development, not a single implementation. Deploy with good-enough data quality, deliver value, improve continuously. Organisations waiting for perfect data quality before deploying AI never deploy and never learn what "good enough" actually means for their specific use cases.

5. Cloud strategy is partnership strategy. Extraction models fail; joint-investment models succeed.

   Organisations structuring cloud relationships as "we rent, you deliver" rather than "we both invest in this platform's success" build dependencies that limit innovation. The best partnerships involve shared investment, aligned incentives, transparent governance and exit flexibility. When both parties have skin in the game, platforms strengthen over time. When one party profits while the other absorbs costs and risks, platforms eventually collapse under misaligned incentives.

Opening

The IT Steering Committee

Samantha sits in the trust's IT steering committee meeting, laptop open to the digital project portfolio dashboard. Seventeen separate initiatives. Each with its own data extract. Each with its own vendor. Each with its own clinical champion arguing for priority funding.

The ED wants AI-powered triage. Radiology wants an imaging analytics platform. The discharge team wants predictive modelling for length of stay. Outpatients want automated appointment reminders. Pathology wants a results-flagging system. All reasonable. All evidence-based. All disconnected.

She pulls up Margaret's care record across three different systems: cardiology at the regional hospital, neurology at the specialist centre, her GP's practice management system. The systems don't talk. They can't share data automatically. Samantha is the integration layer, copying medication lists between systems, explaining to one specialist what another has decided, coordinating appointments that should coordinate themselves.

The irony strikes hard: The trust is building 17 new AI islands when patients need a connected continent. Her mother needs care that connects. Instead, Margaret gets care that requires a daughter with health care expertise to manually integrate what technology promises but can't deliver.

The capital allocation slide appears. Another £4.2 million for "digital transformation". But transformation to what? More sophisticated islands? Better disconnected tools?

Samantha looks at the list again. Seventeen initiatives. None connected to the trust's core EPR. None sharing data with each other. None building on previous investments. Each starting from scratch.

A question forms, uncomfortable and clarifying: What if they stopped adding projects and started building a platform?

The budget vote is called. Samantha abstains. The projects pass anyway. Seventeen disconnected islands, growing.

Field Lesson 1: From Projects to Platform

The Project Accumulation Trap

Seventeen separate digital initiatives. ED AI triage. Radiology imaging analytics. Discharge prediction modelling. Outpatient appointment automation. Pathology results flagging. Each reasonable. Each evidence-based. Each disconnected.

This is the project accumulation trap health care organisations fall into repeatedly. Good intentions, solid business cases, clinical champions, but no platform thinking. Seventeen ways to solve 17 problems independently, starting from scratch each time.

Platform thinking works differently. It asks, does this initiative make the next initiative easier? If the answer is no, you're accumulating projects, not building platforms.

Consider what happened when Samantha's organisation deployed the ED triage tool. It required custom data extraction from the EPR, custom integration with the clinical dashboard, custom training for staff and custom monitoring infrastructure. Six months, £400,000, impressive accuracy scores. Success. Then radiology wanted their imaging analytics platform. Different vendor, same hospital, same EPR. Started from scratch. New data extraction process. New integration approach. New training programme. New monitoring. Another six months, another £400,000. Also successful. The pattern repeated 17 times. Each project delivered value in isolation. None made subsequent projects easier. The integration complexity stayed constant or increased as systems proliferated. That's the signal: When project 15 is as hard as project one, you're not building a platform.

What Platform Thinking Looks Like

Platform thinking inverts the pattern. The first project solves an immediate problem while deliberately building reusable infrastructure. The second project leverages that infrastructure, becoming faster and cheaper than the first. The tenth project is trivial because nine previous projects built the platform it needs.

Kaiser Permanente's multi-year modernisation demonstrates this at scale. Early clinical implementations established core infrastructure—data layer, integration patterns, cloud architecture. Each subsequent application built on and extended that foundation. Later deployments happened faster, cost less, integrated more cleanly. The platform effect compounded. That compounding, where each success makes future success easier, distinguishes platforms from project portfolios.

The test is simple but unforgiving: measure time-to-deployment for your AI initiatives. Plot it over time. If deployment speed increases as you implement more tools, you're building a platform. If it stays constant or slows, you're accumulating projects. The hardest part isn't technical. It's organisational. Project thinking gets rewarded immediately—solve problem, get budget, show ROI, move on. Platform thinking requires different metrics. Instead of "Did we deliver this project on time?" ask "Did this project make the platform stronger?" Instead of "What's the ROI of this tool?" ask "How much faster will the next five tools deploy because this one exists?"

Platform thinking means accepting that early initiatives carry double burden: solve immediate problems while building shared infrastructure. That investment pays off when initiative five costs half what initiative one did. When initiative 10 takes six weeks instead of six months. When integration happens in days, not quarters. But it requires patience, architectural discipline and organisational commitment to value infrastructure investments that don't produce immediate clinical wins. That's why platform thinking is rare in health care despite being standard in technology companies. Health care rewards solving today's problem today. Platforms require solving today's problem while building for tomorrow's.

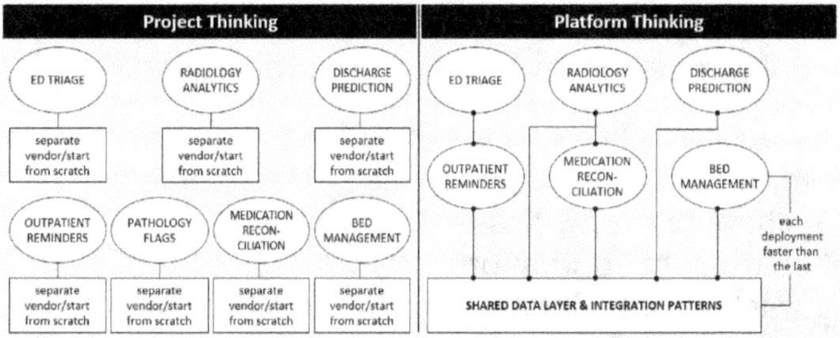

Figure 6. Project thinking restarts from scratch for every deployment. Platform thinking builds a shared data layer so each subsequent deployment is faster than the last.

The critical insight is this: Platforms emerge from disciplined success, not from architectural planning that precedes value delivery. You cannot design the perfect platform in year one. You discover it by solving real problems, learning what's reusable, extracting patterns and deliberately building infrastructure that subsequent problems can draw on. Each solved problem becomes a platform building block if you extract the lessons and create the reusable components.

Field Lesson 2: Infrastructure Investment Discipline

The Infrastructure-First Trap

The infrastructure-first trap looks rational on paper. Spend three years building perfect data architecture. Establish comprehensive governance. Design elegant integration frameworks. Deploy cloud infrastructure at scale. Then, once foundations are solid, roll out applications that build on all this preparation.

Except clinical problems evolve faster than infrastructure projects. Stakeholders change. Requirements shift. Technology advances. Three years is forever in health care operations. By the time the perfect infrastructure arrives, it's addressing yesterday's challenges with assumptions that no longer hold.

Estonia's Counterexample

Estonia offers a counterexample that seems to contradict "deliver value quarterly" until you examine what actually happened.

Estonia's X-Road infrastructure project ran from 2001 to 2008. Seven years building the secure data exchange layer that would eventually support the national electronic health record, digital prescriptions and hundreds of other government services. That timeline sounds like exactly the kind of long-term infrastructure investment that paralyses organisations.

But X-Road delivered incremental value throughout those seven years. It didn't wait until 2008 to launch applications. The infrastructure enabled government services progressively: first simple data exchanges, then more complex transactions, building capability and proving value continuously. By the time the health record launched, X-Road had already processed millions of transactions for other government functions. The platform was battle-tested, not theoretical.

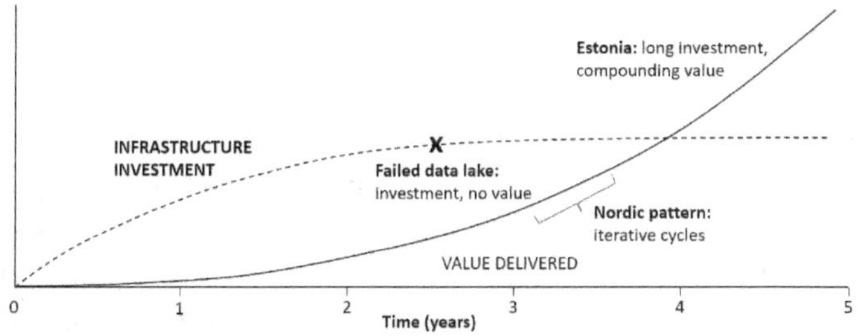

Figure 7. Estonia's long investment compounds. The Nordic pattern—iterative cycles—delivers continuous value. The failed data lake: investment with no value delivered.

That discipline—build infrastructure that enables quarterly wins while supporting long-term vision—distinguishes successful platform investments from infrastructure projects that consume resources without delivering value. Estonia's patience was architectural, not operational. They took seven years to build foundational infrastructure correctly, but that infrastructure enabled incremental value delivery from early stages.

The results validate the approach. X-Road now processes 2.2 billion transactions annually. Estonia achieved 100% digital health records and 99% digital prescriptions. The Estonian Health Insurance Fund operates at 0.9% administrative costs—a fraction of comparable systems elsewhere—because infrastructure was built to compound efficiency over time.

The Nordic Pattern

Nordic health care systems demonstrate the same pattern repeatedly. Denmark's Sundhed.dk launched in 2003 and has evolved continuously for over two decades through systematic four-to-five-year enhancement cycles. Finland's Kanta platform represents 20 years of ecosystem development, not a single implementation. Both deliver value quarterly while investing in infrastructure that compounds over decades.

The false choice between “deliver quickly” and “build foundations” paralyses organisations that haven't learnt this lesson. The right answer is both. Solve immediate clinical problems using existing infrastructure, where possible, while systematically extracting reusable components and patterns that make subsequent problems easier. Each clinical win should strengthen the platform. Each infrastructure investment should enable near-term value.

The metric that matters: time between infrastructure investment and value delivery. If you deploy infrastructure and wait months before applications use it, your timing is wrong. Infrastructure should enable value within weeks, not quarters. Applications should inform infrastructure design immediately, not eventually.

Samantha's organisation learnt this when they proposed building a comprehensive data lake before deploying any analytics. Eighteen months. £2 million. Promise of future capability. The chief financial officer's (CFO) question cut through: "What value do we get in month six?" The honest answer, "Capability to build tools that deliver value in month 19," killed the proposal. The revised approach: deploy analytics for one specific use case in six weeks. Build exactly the data infrastructure that use case requires. Extract reusable patterns. Deploy analytics for use case two in four weeks, building on the infrastructure from use case one. Continue. Each deployment strengthens infrastructure. Each infrastructure investment enables faster deployment. The platform emerges from success, not from planning.

Field Lesson 3: Integration Architecture Determines Success

Why Brilliant AI Dies in Integration

Brilliant algorithms fail in health care for a simple reason: They can't integrate with clinical workflow. The AI achieves 95% accuracy in testing. Clinicians love the prototype. Then deployment reveals the problem: Getting data into the system and recommendations into clinician hands requires custom integration that nobody budgeted for, architected properly or understood the complexity of.

NHS Fife's experience with the Morse EPR integration demonstrates what success looks like. The Morse EPR integrated with the Orion Health portal to eliminate duplicate appointment entries and give clinicians complete patient views across community and acute systems. That integration work, not the EPR software itself, created value. Without reliable data flow between systems, even sophisticated technology delivers zero clinical benefit.

The NHS's digital transformation investment recognises this reality explicitly. Integration costs will exceed technology costs by three to five times for most implementations. Organisations treating integration as an afterthought—"We'll figure that out in phase two"—repeat the 80 – 92% pilot failure rate from earlier chapters. Those planning for integration complexity from day one build platforms where subsequent integrations become progressively easier.

Integration-First Thinking

Integration-first thinking looks different from technology-first thinking. Technology-first asks, "Which AI tool solves this problem?" Integration-first asks, "How does the solution fit into existing clinical workflow, and what infrastructure changes enable that fit?" Consider sepsis detection. Technology-first thinking selects the best algorithm, proves accuracy in testing then discovers the challenge: The algorithm needs real-time lab results, vital signs, medication data and clinical notes to function. But labs use one system, vitals come from monitoring devices, medications flow through pharmacy systems and notes live in the EPR. Integrating these data streams requires custom work for each source. The algorithm is ready. The integration isn't. Integration-first thinking inverts this. Before selecting algorithms, map data flows. What systems hold the data? How do they expose it? What's the API architecture? Where does latency occur? Then design integration architecture that makes real-time data available through standard patterns. Multiple algorithms can use that infrastructure once built. The integration complexity decreases as you deploy more tools, not increases.

The NHS Fife example succeeded because integration architecture was explicit and central. The Morse EPR and Orion Health portal teams designed integration interfaces together, not sequentially. They established data standards, API contracts and synchronisation patterns before building features. That upfront investment paid off as new capabilities deployed faster because integration patterns were reusable.

The practical approach: Pick one AI use case. Build it fully integrated into clinical workflow. Extract every integration pattern as reusable infrastructure. Document what worked, what didn't and where complexity hides. Then deploy use case two, measuring how much integration effort decreased because patterns from use case one are reusable. If integration effort stays constant, your patterns aren't reusable enough. If it decreases, you're building a platform.

This requires organisational changes beyond technology. Traditional procurement treats each technology purchase independently. Platform procurement considers how each purchase affects integration complexity. Will this vendor's API architecture fit our patterns? Does this tool reduce or increase integration burden on subsequent tools? Finance must understand that integration costs aren't waste; they're infrastructure investment. The first integration into a new data source is expensive. The tenth integration into that same source should cost a fraction of the first.

Field Lesson 4: Partnership Models That Work

Cloud Strategy as Partnership Decision

Cloud strategy isn't a technology decision; it's a partnership decision. The technical architecture matters, but the relationship structure determines whether cloud investments strengthen your platform or create vendor dependencies that limit innovation.

Traditional vendor-customer models fail in cloud contexts because interests misalign immediately. The vendor profits from consumption—more storage, more compute, more services purchased. The customer seeks efficiency, delivering more value with less infrastructure cost. This fundamental tension ensures one party wins at the other's expense. That's a zero-sum game where long-term partnerships can't survive.

The NHS Palantir Federated Data Platform contract provides a test case for whether health care can structure cloud partnerships differently. By 2028/29, all NHS acute, community and mental health providers would use the Federated Data Program (FDP), making the partnership model absolutely critical to success.

Four Elements That Distinguish Partnership from Extraction

The difference between successful partnerships and extraction models comes down to four specific structural elements:

"Shared investment" means both parties have capital at risk. When only the customer pays and only the vendor profits, incentives misalign. Successful partnerships involve vendors investing in platform development, implementation support and outcome achievement, not just selling licences. Kaiser Permanente's cloud relationships work because vendors invested in Kaiser's success, not just in selling capacity. That shared risk creates shared commitment to outcomes. "Aligned incentives" means success metrics benefit both parties simultaneously. If vendor revenue increases while customer costs rise, the partnership is extractive. If both parties benefit from improved efficiency, reduced costs or better outcomes, incentives align. This requires creative commercial structures—outcome-based pricing, shared savings models or revenue tied to platform adoption and value delivery rather than infrastructure consumption.

“Governance transparency” means decision rights are explicit and balanced. Who controls roadmap priorities? How are technical decisions made? What happens when interests conflict? Successful partnerships establish clear governance from the start. Opaque governance where vendors hold asymmetric information or decision power creates extraction opportunities.

“Exit flexibility” means genuine partnerships include exit provisions that protect both parties without creating lock-in. The customer must be able to terminate without prohibitive switching costs. The vendor must be compensated fairly for investments made. Successful partnerships make exit possible but rarely attractive because ongoing value exceeds exit alternatives. Lock-in through proprietary formats, exorbitant switching costs or contractual penalties signals extraction, not partnership.

The Procurement Shift

Traditional Requests for Proposals (RFPs) focus on technical capabilities and price. Platform-oriented procurement evaluates partnership structure. How does the vendor make money? Do their incentives align with our efficiency goals? What governance protects our interests? Can we exit if the partnership fails?

Finance teams struggle with this because it looks more expensive initially. Partnerships with shared investment and aligned incentives cost more upfront than traditional licences. But extraction models cost far more long-term. The licence is cheap. The lock-in is expensive. Organisations must learn to value partnership structure over initial price—the same dual-win thinking that applies to consulting relationships applies to cloud partnerships.

Framework Close: Operating System Readiness

Before approving your next digital transformation budget, the leadership team should be able to answer four questions clearly. If they can't, you're funding projects, not building a platform.

What's the one clinical problem we could solve in six to eight weeks using existing infrastructure, and how would solving it create reusable components for the next problem?

Does our governance model enable data sharing with clear rules and transparent access, or does it create six-month approval processes that amount to paralysis?

How many of our current AI initiatives share common data infrastructure and integration patterns, and does each new tool make the next one easier or harder to deploy?

Can we point to clinical outcomes, operational improvements or patient experience gains within 90 days of any infrastructure investment, and if not, are we building the wrong infrastructure?

Back to Samantha

Three weeks after the IT steering committee meeting, Samantha requests a meeting with the trust's chief information officer (CIO). She brings data: the 17 initiatives, their budgets, their timelines and their integration status. None connected. Total budget: £8.4 million over three years. Total integration plan: "to be determined".

"What if we tried something different?" she asks. "Not smaller, different."

She proposes using £400,000—less than 5% of the planned digital transformation budget—to solve one specific problem in eight weeks: discharge delays in elderly care. Not build infrastructure. Not plan integration. Just solve one problem that costs the trust over £2 million annually in bed-day waste.

"Use our existing EPR. Use our existing data. Build something clinicians can actually use in workflow. Show it works. Then expand." The CIO is sceptical. "That's not transformation. That's a pilot."

"No," Samantha says. "A pilot is disconnected. This is the first building block of a platform. If it works, the next problem uses the same infrastructure. And the problem after that. Each solution makes the next one cheaper and faster. That's a platform."

She pulls up Estonia's X-Road on her laptop. "They spent seven years building infrastructure before launching applications. We can't do that. No board would approve it. But we can solve real problems while building infrastructure that makes subsequent problems easier. Platform thinking, not project thinking."

The CIO asks the question Samantha expected: "What's the Monday morning action?"

"Form a small team. One clinical informatics lead. One developer who knows our EPR's API. One process improvement analyst. Give them eight weeks and £400,000. If they solve discharge delays and build reusable components, we have proof of concept. If they fail, we've spent less than one of our 17 disconnected projects."

The CIO agrees to propose it to the executive committee. Not as replacement for the 17 initiatives but as a different approach to test alongside them. Samantha thinks about Margaret that evening. Her mother's care still requires a daughter as integration layer. But maybe, if platform thinking took root, patients five years from now wouldn't need technical expertise in their families. Maybe systems would finally connect the way health care always should have.

Remember the Five Things

These aren't five separate infrastructure decisions. They're a connected system, and the sequence matters as much as the substance.

1. Platform thinking beats project thinking.

   But only when platforms emerge from solved problems, not from architectural plans that precede value delivery. The test is whether each new initiative makes the next one easier. If deployment speed isn't increasing, you're accumulating projects regardless of what you call them. Kaiser's $1.5 billion in annual savings came from this compounding effect, not from superior algorithms.

2. Infrastructure investment earns its place through quarterly value delivery.

   Estonia and the Nordics show that even long-term platform investments must prove themselves incrementally. Infrastructure that can't show tangible clinical or operational value within 90 days is probably the wrong infrastructure or the wrong sequencing. The data lake that takes 18 months before anyone can use it has already failed regardless of how elegant its architecture.

3. Integration architecture determines success.

   Even brilliant AI delivers zero value if clinicians can't access it in workflow. The three to five times cost multiplier for integration isn't waste; it's the real cost of making technology work in health care. Organisations that plan for this from day one build platforms where each subsequent integration becomes progressively easier. Those treating integration as an afterthought repeat the 80 – 92% failure rate indefinitely.

4. Data quality improves through use, not through waiting.

   The Nordic pattern—deploy with good-enough quality for specific use cases, then improve through systematic cycles—resolves the paralysis that traps organisations in "data isn't ready yet". Twenty years of Finnish and Danish experience show that data quality is an outcome of systematic deployment, not a prerequisite for it.

5. Cloud partnership structure matters more than cloud technical architecture.

   Shared investment, aligned incentives, transparent governance and exit flexibility distinguish partnerships that strengthen over time from extraction models that create dependency. The same dual-win principle applies here as with consulting: The question isn't whether to use external partners but whether the relationship builds organisational capability or replaces it.

The operating system provides the platform. Chapter 5 addresses what makes it intelligent—the ontological understanding that teaches AI what health care concepts actually mean, how they relate to each other and why a cardiologist sees connections in "heart failure" that an algorithm processing text strings cannot.

Chapter 5
The Ontology Layer

Making AI Understand Health Care's Complexity

Key message: AI needs more than data. It needs understanding. Ontologies teach AI what health care concepts mean and how they relate to each other. Without this shared understanding, sophisticated algorithms remain fundamentally disconnected from clinical reality. The gap between having data and comprehending data determines whether AI transforms care or merely adds complexity. You don't need perfect ontologies to start. Even basic standardisation delivers immediate value. The sophistication comes from consistency over time, not complexity on day one.

If You Read Nothing Else, Remember These Five Things

1. Standard vocabularies solve one problem but create another.

   Systematized Nomenclature of Medicine—Clinical Terms (SNOMED CT), Logical Observation Identifiers Names and Codes (LOINC) and RxNorm each provide structured ways to describe clinical concepts. But they don't naturally talk to each other. One system calls a medication "Metoprolol Succinate ER", another "Metoprolol XL" and a third, "Toprol-XL." Same drug. Three names. No automatic recognition. Standard vocabularies are necessary but insufficient; you need ontologies that understand relationships, not just labels.

2. World models matter more than large language models for health care.

   LLMs manipulate language brilliantly; they generate coherent text, summarise documents and answer questions. But health care needs systems that understand how the physical world actually works: how medications interact with physiology, how conditions progress over time, how treatments affect outcomes. World models simulate reality. That's the difference between an AI that sounds intelligent and one that understands medicine.

3. Digital twins are ontologies in action.

   A digital twin is a living model that understands what data means and how elements relate. Patient-level twins simulate individual health trajectories. Hospital-level twins model operations. Population-level twins predict disease patterns. The NHS is piloting personalised digital heart twins. Mayo Clinic and Siemens are building AI-enhanced cardiovascular twins. This isn't future technology; it's operational today in organisations that built the ontology foundation first.

4. Simulate in digital before deploying in physical.

   Waymo doesn't train autonomous vehicles by letting them crash into things and learning from mistakes. They simulate millions of scenarios digitally, test responses, refine models and then deploy to the physical world with confidence. Health care should work the same way. Simulate patient journeys before rolling out new care pathways. Test AI interventions in digital twins before deploying to real patients. The digital world becomes your safe learning environment.

5. Clinical involvement in ontology design is non-negotiable.

   Engineering thinking alone produces technically elegant systems that don't match clinical reality. Clinical thinking alone produces workflows that can't scale. Clinicians must define how AI understands their workflows, what relationships matter and which distinctions are clinically meaningful versus administratively arbitrary. Organisations that build ontologies without clinical involvement build expensive systems nobody uses.

Opening

The Pharmacy Call

The pharmacy calls Samantha at 4:47 pm on Friday afternoon.

"We need clarification on your mother's prescription. The cardiologist prescribed Metoprolol Succinate ER. Your GP's system shows Metoprolol XL. We have Toprol-XL in stock. Are these the same medication?"

Samantha closes her office door. Of course they're the same. Any pharmacist knows this immediately. But the three "intelligent" health care systems managing her mother's care don't.

She pulls up Margaret's records across the three portals she now manages daily. The cardiologist's notes discuss heart failure using precise clinical terminology. The memory clinic describes vascular dementia with equal rigour. The GP's system tries to integrate both, creating a patchwork of references that don't align.

If systems can't understand that Metoprolol Succinate ER and Metoprolol XL are the same drug, how can they understand the relationship between her mother's conditions? How can AI predict which medications might interact, which symptoms signal deterioration and which interventions might help?

The AI doesn't lack data. Her mother's health history spans three decades across multiple systems. The AI lacks understanding—information without meaning, labels without relationships, data without ontology.

Samantha confirms with the pharmacy that yes, these are the same medication. She updates the spreadsheet she maintains manually—her own desperate attempt to create what the systems should provide automatically: a unified understanding of her mother's care. The irony isn't lost on her. She's become the human ontology layer, the integration point the technology should have been.

Field Lesson 1: What Ontology Actually Means

The Standards Paradox

Start with the problem everyone recognises: Health care is drowning in standards, yet somehow nothing connects properly.

SNOMED CT contains over 300,000 medical concepts: diagnoses, procedures, findings, anatomical structures. It's the world's most comprehensive clinical terminology, developed by an international consortium, implemented across dozens of countries. LOINC provides 95,000+ terms for laboratory tests and clinical observations. RxNorm standardises medication names across 13 source vocabularies, updated monthly by the US National Library of Medicine. These aren't small efforts. They represent decades of work by thousands of experts. Yet here's what actually happens: A patient presents with chest pain. The ED codes it one way in SNOMED CT. The lab results come back through LOINC. The prescribed medications flow through

RxNorm. Three different systems, three different organisational schemes, three different ways of representing medical reality. Each is internally coherent. Each is technically sophisticated. And each requires extensive mapping to communicate with the others. The Systematized Nomenclature of Medicine, Logic, Observation and Representation (SOLOR) project, an initiative led by the Veterans Administration, attempts to integrate SNOMED CT, LOINC and RxNorm into a unified description-logic-based system. It's necessary because even having all three standards doesn't automatically create interoperability. Standards define vocabularies. Ontologies define understanding.

Here's the distinction that matters: A vocabulary says, "These are the approved terms". An ontology says, "This is what the terms mean and how they relate". Vocabulary gives you consistency. Ontology gives you comprehension.

From Labels to Relationships

Think about the Metoprolol example. RxNorm knows that Metoprolol Succinate ER, Metoprolol XL and Toprol-XL are related. It has mappings. But knowing they're related isn't the same as understanding they're the same drug in different formulations. That understanding—"same active ingredient, extended release, different branding"—requires ontological knowledge, not just terminological mapping. Now scale that problem. A hospital system isn't trying to understand one medication. It's trying to understand thousands of medications, millions of lab results, billions of clinical observations and how they all relate to each other in the context of individual patients with complex, interacting conditions. Without ontologies, you get systems that know a lot but understand little.

The question organisations must answer is, "What does your data model look like, reflecting your business?" Not which standard should you adopt; you'll adopt multiple. But what's the organisational understanding that connects them?

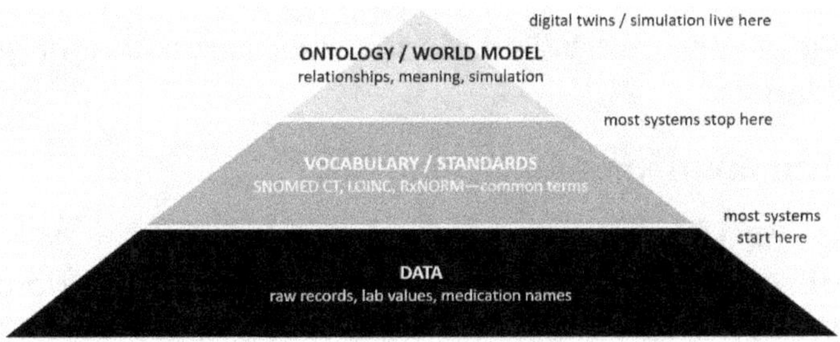

Figure 8. Most systems start at data and stop at vocabulary/standards. The ontology/world model layer—where digital twins and simulation live—is where most stop short.

The Operating System chapter, Chapter 4, discussed data foundations. This is the layer above that. Data governance ensures quality. Ontologies ensure meaning. Both are necessary. Neither is sufficient alone. That distinction between having data and understanding data is what separates systems that describe health care from systems that comprehend it. Most organisations begin with basic SNOMED CT mapping for one clinical concept: diagnoses for sepsis, medication classes for polypharmacy alerts or lab result patterns for early warning systems. Pick one concept that matters clinically and appears frequently. Map it consistently across your systems. That single standardised concept delivering value in one decision proves the approach works. Sophistication comes from repeating this process systematically, not from attempting comprehensive mapping on day one.

Field Lesson 2: World Models over Large Language Models

The Fundamental Distinction

Demis Hassabis, CEO of Google DeepMind, made an observation that cuts through the AI hype: World models matter more than LLMs for health care. World models simulate reality. LLMs manipulate language. Large language models have transformed how we interact with information. They write impressively coherent text, translate between languages, summarise documents and answer questions with apparent fluency. ChatGPT, Gemini, Claude—these systems demonstrate remarkable linguistic capability. They've mastered the patterns of human communication. But health care doesn't need systems that talk about medicine impressively. Health care needs systems that understand how medicine actually works. A world model represents how physical reality functions, capturing cause and effect, temporal dynamics, spatial relationships and mechanistic connections. It simulates what happens when you change a variable because it understands the underlying system, not just how people describe it.

Consider diabetes management. A large language model (LLM) can eloquently describe diabetes complications, treatment options and monitoring recommendations. It can synthesise guidelines, generate patient education materials and answer questions about medication interactions. All valuable capabilities. But it's operating at the level of description, not understanding. A world model of diabetes would simulate how glucose levels respond to insulin dosing, how dietary changes affect blood sugar over time and how exercise impacts insulin sensitivity in specific individuals. It would model the physiological processes, not just the language people use to discuss them. The difference determines whether AI can predict outcomes, optimise treatments and personalise interventions or just document care eloquently.

Digital Twins: World Models in Action

Digital twins are world models applied to health care. They're virtual representations of physical entities that simulate behaviour, not just describe it. Patient-level digital twins model individual health. The NHS is piloting personalised digital heart twins that use imaging, sensor data and wearable information to predict cardiovascular disease progression for specific individuals. These aren't general risk calculators. They're patient-specific simulations that understand how that person's unique physiology responds to interventions.

Hospital-level digital twins model operations. Nearly 40% of large hospitals now deploy digital twins for resource optimisation, surgical planning and care coordination. Duke University's digital twin programme uses simulation to test different scenarios before implementation, understanding how changes will ripple through the system rather than discovering problems after deployment.

Population-level digital twins model community health patterns, simulating how disease spreads through populations, how interventions affect outcomes at scale and where resources should be allocated for maximum impact. The difference between a dashboard showing population statistics and a digital twin simulating population dynamic is the difference between description and understanding. These require what Hassabis calls "macro-meso-micro perspectives"—different ontologies at each level. Patient-level twins need detailed physiological models. Hospital-level twins need operational and workflow models. Population-level twins need epidemiological and resource models. The ontology that works at one level doesn't automatically scale to another. This is where health care differs from domains like autonomous vehicles. Waymo needs one primary level of ontology—the vehicle's relationship to its immediate environment. Health care needs nested ontologies that work across multiple scales simultaneously. A patient exists within a care team, which operates within a hospital, which serves a population. Each level requires its own understanding, and all must connect coherently. The technical term for this is "ontological interoperability" —not just data talking to data but understanding connecting to understanding.

Hassabis offers one more insight worth carrying forward: "If you can simulate something, you've understood it." That's the test. Can your AI simulate a patient's response to treatment? Can it simulate workflow changes? Can it simulate disease progression? If not, you have description, not understanding. And description alone doesn't transform care. Ninety-day ontology wins: Organisations don't need complete world models to start delivering value. Pick one repeating clinical decision that happens hundreds of times daily—antibiotic selection for sepsis, discharge readiness assessment or fall risk evaluation. Map the relationships that decision depends on: which labs matter, how vital signs interact, what medication contraindications exist. Build just enough ontology to improve that one decision. When accuracy increases or decision time decreases measurably within 90 days, you've proven the approach works. Then expand systematically, building ontological understanding incrementally rather than attempting comprehensive modelling upfront.

Field Lesson 3: Connecting Digital and Physical Worlds

The Waymo Principle

Vincent Vanhoucke, distinguished engineer at Waymo, described their development approach clearly: There's a digital world and a physical world. They practise simulating the digital world and then implement in the physical world.

The key insight is the absence of real-time dependency. Waymo doesn't train autonomous vehicles by connecting them to cloud-based intelligence that tells them what to do moment-by-moment. That would be dangerous and impractical. Instead, they simulate millions of scenarios in the digital world, train models on those simulations, verify performance and then deploy self-contained systems to the physical world. Learn in simulation. Deploy with confidence. The physical system operates independently, but it's been trained against digital truth.

Health Care's Current Pattern and the Alternative

The current typical pattern in health care is to develop an AI algorithm, run a small pilot in a controlled setting, discover problems during real-world deployment and iterate based on what breaks. It's expensive, risky and slow. Every failure happens on a real patient or in a real clinical workflow. Every iteration costs time and trust. The alternative: Build digital twins of patient journeys, simulate interventions, test AI systems against those simulations, refine until performance is reliable and then deploy to physical care delivery. The simulation becomes the safe learning environment. Reality is where you apply what you've learnt, not where you discover what doesn't work.

Some organisations are already doing this. Siemens Healthineers and Mayo Clinic are developing AI-enhanced cardiovascular twins that simulate patient-specific responses before implementing interventions. The inHEART system—FDA clearance March 2024—generates 3D cardiac models enabling simulation-based treatment planning with results showing 60% reduction in procedure times and 38% decrease in recurrence rates. That's not iterative trial-and-error. That's simulation-validated intervention.

The FDA itself is moving in this direction. In January 2025, they issued draft guidance encouraging digital twin simulations in regulatory submissions for medical devices and clinical trials, recognising them as valid tools for assessing safety and effectiveness. They're acknowledging what engineering fields have known for decades: Simulation reduces risk when done rigorously.

Understanding Simulation Limitations

Simulations are powerful but not infallible. They fail when underlying assumptions are wrong, when training data doesn't represent real-world variation or when rare edge cases aren't modelled. The inHEART results are impressive because they focused on specific cardiac procedures with well-understood physics. Simulations work best for systems with known rules and measurable variables. They struggle with emergent behaviours, social dynamics and situations involving significant uncertainty.

The critical caveat: The ontologies underlying the digital twins must be correct. If your simulation doesn't understand the relationships between variables, it produces beautiful visualisations of nonsense. If your patient twin doesn't model physiology accurately, its predictions mislead rather than inform. The quality of simulation is bounded by the quality of ontological understanding.

Always validate simulation outputs against real-world outcomes before trusting them for critical decisions. Start with simple simulations of well-understood processes, measure accuracy rigorously and expand scope only when validation proves reliability. When simulation results contradict clinical judgement, investigate the discrepancy. Either the simulation is wrong or clinical assumptions need updating.

Field Lesson 4: Clinical Involvement in Ontology Design

Partnership Done Right

In April 2025, Burjeel Holdings partnered with Hippocratic AI for agentic AI capability achieving 99.38% clinical accuracy across 15+ languages. The strategic decision was to partner rather than build. But Burjeel's clinical teams defined requirements first. "What capabilities do we need? What must the AI understand? Which relationships matter in our workflows?" Then they evaluated build-buy-partner options from a position of clarity.

That's clinical involvement done right. Not "build it, then show us". But clinicians and engineers designing together, validating together, refining together.

Why Both Perspectives Are Essential

Engineering thinking and clinical thinking solve different problems. Engineers optimise systems, reduce complexity and create elegance. Clinicians navigate ambiguity, balance competing priorities and make decisions under uncertainty. Health care needs both.

An engineer might define "patient deterioration" with clean thresholds: temperature above X, blood pressure below Y. Elegant. Computable. Wrong. A clinician knows deterioration is contextual. The same vital signs mean different things in different patients. Pattern matters more than absolute values. That contextual understanding must be encoded in the ontology.

Conversely, “I know it when I see it” is valuable but computationally useless. The engineer’s contribution is making implicit understanding explicit and translatable.

Vendors can accelerate development substantially if relationships are structured correctly. The best vendors bring ontology expertise from solving similar problems elsewhere. But vendors become problematic when they drive your show rather than support it. The question to ask is, “Can you adapt your ontology to our workflows, or must we change workflows to match yours?” The first half suggests partnership. The second suggests problems.

Three Clarity Points

Three things matter when designing the clinical-engineering collaboration for ontology work. First, what clinical understanding is non-negotiable versus adaptable? Some relationships are clinically essential. Others are process-dependent. Know which is which. Second, who owns the ontology long-term? If vendors control updates, you’ve outsourced your organisational understanding. Third, how does the ontology evolve? Clinical practice changes. Your ontology must evolve with your organisation, not remain frozen. The build-buy-partner decision is actually a control question. Many organisations partner initially with phased internal capability building. Start with vendor expertise, learn from implementation and gradually develop internal ontology management. It's a maturity curve, not a binary choice. The same principle from Chapter 3's consulting discussion applies: The best relationships build organisational muscle, not reliance.

Framework Close: Ontology Readiness

Four questions determine whether your organisation is ready to build the ontology layer that makes AI meaningful:

1. Do our systems share a common language for clinical concepts, not just standards implementation but actual shared understanding? Can a diagnosis in one system connect to lab results in another and medications in a third without manual intervention? If humans are the integration layer, your ontology doesn't exist yet.

2. Can we simulate patient journeys before deploying AI interventions, not in theory but today? Do we have digital twin capability, even in pilot form? Organisations with mature ontologies can simulate. Organisations without them can only deploy and hope.

3. Are clinicians involved in defining how AI understands our workflows, not consulted after design, not trained after deployment but involved in ontology design itself? If ontology is viewed as an IT project rather than a clinical knowledge project, you're building for technical elegance, not clinical utility.

4. Is our build-buy-partner strategy for ontology capabilities intentional or accidental? Most organisations will partner initially, build capability gradually and then manage their ontologies with vendor tools rather than vendor services. But the path requires intention, not drift.

Back to Samantha

Three weeks after the medication name confusion, Samantha sits in a planning session about the trust's digital twin initiative. The vendor is enthusiastic, the slides impressive, the promises ambitious. They'll create digital twins of patient journeys, optimise care pathways and predict complications before they occur.

"What's the ontology here?" Samantha asks.

The room goes quiet. The vendor hesitates.

"We use SNOMED CT for diagnoses, LOINC for lab values, RxNorm for medications," they say. "All the standard vocabularies." "That's not what I asked," Samantha says gently. "Where's the ontological understanding? How does your system know that my mother's heart failure and vascular dementia are related conditions that influence each other's treatment? How does it understand that what looks like deterioration in one patient might be baseline in another? What relationships does your world model actually model?"

The vendor's response is careful. "We can work with your clinical teams to define those relationships. That's part of the implementation process."

Exactly. Not "We've solved this" but "We can help you solve it". That's the difference between a vendor partner and a vendor driver.

Later, walking back to her office, Samantha feels something she hasn't felt in months about the trust's AI initiatives: clarity. Not about having solutions. About understanding the problem. The gap between data and meaning is wider than she thought, but now she knows why. And knowing why means it's addressable. The medication name problem that frustrated her makes sense now. The systems have vocabularies but not ontologies. They have terms but not understanding. They know what "Metoprolol Succinate ER" means in isolation but not how it relates to other formulations, other medications or other conditions.

Building that understanding is feasible. Hard, yes. Time-consuming, certainly. But feasible. The path is visible: Define critical relationships with clinical input, structure them formally, simulate before deploying, evolve based on outcomes, partner where appropriate, build where necessary and maintain control throughout.

She's not naive. This will take years, not months. Quarterly wins building toward transformation. But years with direction beat decades of drift.

Remember the Five Things

These aren't five separate technical concepts. They're a progression, each building on what came before, each making the next possible.

1. Standard vocabularies are essential.

   SNOMED CT, LOINC, RxNorm provide consistency. But ontologies provide understanding. One gives you common terms. The other gives you meaning and relationships. The Metoprolol problem—same drug, three names, no recognition—exists because systems have vocabularies without ontologies. Start with one clinical concept mapped consistently across your systems. That single standardised concept proving value in one decision is enough to prove the approach works.

2. World models matter more than language models.

   Health care needs systems that understand how medicine works, not just how to talk about it impressively. The test Hassabis offers—"If you can simulate something, you've understood it"—

is the dividing line between AI that describes health care and AI that comprehends it. Description alone doesn't transform care.

3. Digital twins are ontologies in action.

   Patient-level twins simulating individual health, hospital-level twins modelling operations, population-level twins predicting outcomes. They're operational today in organisations that built the ontology layer first. The inHEART system's 60% reduction in procedure times and 38% decrease in recurrence rates show what's possible when simulation replaces trial-and-error. But simulation quality is bounded by ontological accuracy; beautiful visualisations of wrong relationships produce beautiful nonsense.

4. Simulate in digital before deploying in physical.

   The Waymo principle applies: Learn in simulation; deploy with confidence. Every failure that happens in simulation is a failure that doesn't happen to a real patient. But simulation has limits; it works best for well-understood systems with measurable variables and must always be validated against real-world outcomes before being trusted for critical decisions.

5. Clinical involvement in ontology design is non-negotiable.

   Engineers structure knowledge computationally. Clinicians define what knowledge matters. Together they build ontologies that reflect reality while remaining technically implementable. The build-buy-partner decision is really a control question, and the same principle from Chapter 3 applies: The best relationships build organisational muscle, not reliance.

The operating system provides the platform. Ontologies make it intelligent. Chapter 6 addresses the question that follows naturally: Now that we can build systems that understand health care, how do humans and AI actually work together? The answer—augmentation, not replacement—is where the book's central question becomes most personal. Samantha thinks about Dr Rahman finally being able to look at patients instead of screens. She thinks about Margaret asking about her prognosis and her cardiologist reaching across to take her hand. Some things AI can enhance. Some things remain irreducibly human. The next chapter explores where the line falls.

Chapter 6
The Augmentation Playbook

Human-AI Collaboration That Actually Works

Key message: AI reveals what makes humans irreplaceable. When machines handle documentation, pattern recognition and routine analysis, clinicians focus on what only humans can provide: clinical judgement, patient relationships, ethical reasoning and context integration. The goal isn't replacement; it's humans upgraded through partnership. But augmentation demands calibration: trust without over-reliance, autonomy without abandonment, efficiency without erosion of expertise.

If You Read Nothing Else, Remember These Five Things

1. AI reveals the human

   When machines handle what machines do best, what remains is distinctly human: judgement, empathy, ethical reasoning and the ability to integrate complex context. AI also reveals problems that existed before AI arrived: documentation as checkbox exercise, clinicians drowning in administrative burden. The technology doesn't create these problems. It exposes them by demonstrating how much "clinical work" was actually routine data processing.

2. Calibration matters more than capability.

   The challenge isn't making AI smarter. It's teaching clinicians when to trust it, when to question it and when to override it. Over-trust leads to cognitive offloading and automation bias. Under-trust leads to expensive systems nobody uses. The middle path requires transparency, feedback loops and, most importantly, cognitive space for the deliberation that builds appropriate trust.

3. Agentic AI changes everything.

   Current AI responds to prompts. The next generation takes initiative, operates autonomously and acts to achieve goals with limited oversight. UC San Diego's COMPOSER system cut sepsis deaths by 17% by monitoring 150 live data points and alerting clinical teams without being asked. Gartner predicts agentic AI will rise from less than 1% of enterprise applications in 2024 to 33% by 2028. Health care needs to be ready and most isn't.

4. Engagement beats approval.

   The best human-AI partnerships aren't about clinicians reviewing and signing off on AI outputs. They're about dialogue: clinicians correcting, contextualising, questioning and providing feedback that improves the system over time. Approval treats clinicians as quality control bottlenecks. Engagement treats them as collaborators whose judgement makes the AI better.

5. Create time for thinking.

   AI's highest value isn't speed; it's creating cognitive space for the clinical reasoning that only humans can provide. If the answer to "What will clinicians do with the time saved?" is "See more patients", you've missed the point. The goal is room for judgement, relationship-building, ethical reasoning and complex problem-solving. These activities take time. AI should create it.

Opening

The Cardiology Appointment

Dr Hassan's practice implemented ambient documentation three months ago. Samantha accompanies her mother Margaret to a routine cardiology appointment, expecting the familiar choreography: warm greeting, immediate pivot to computer, typing while questioning, eyes on screen while Margaret describes her chest tightness.

Today feels different.

Dr Hassan sets his phone on the desk, the app recording, and gives Margaret his full attention. For the first time in years, he looks at her. Really looks. He notices the slight breathlessness when she speaks, how she touches her chest, the flicker of worry when Samantha squeezes her hand.

The AI captures everything—symptoms, timing, severity, Margaret's description of "like an elephant sitting on my chest"—while Dr Hassan maintains eye contact, nods and asks follow-up questions that emerge from genuine listening rather than checklist completion.

Then Margaret asks the question she's been holding: "How much time do I have?"

The ambient documentation continues recording. But Dr Hassan reaches across the desk and takes Margaret's hand. The room becomes smaller, quieter. He speaks about the uncertainty of prognoses, the variability of disease progression, the balance between honest realism and sustaining hope. He acknowledges her fear. He validates Samantha's presence. He creates space for the conversation Margaret actually needs.

The AI captures the words. But it cannot capture this—the weight of held hands, the cadence of difficult truth delivered with compassion, the micro-expressions that signal understanding or the clinical judgement about when facts matter less than presence. As they leave, Margaret tells Samantha she felt heard. Not processed. Heard.

Samantha notices something else. Dr Hassan's notes appear in the system before they reach the car park. Complete, structured, accurate. He didn't stay late tonight entering documentation. The technology freed him to be more human, not less.

But she also noticed Margaret's slight confusion at the beginning of the visit—the invisible listener, the phone on the desk, the sense of being observed by something she couldn't see. Trust, Samantha realises, is earned through transparency and maintained through competence. Both matter. So does explicit patient consent—explaining what's being recorded, how AI will use it and giving patients genuine choice about whether to participate.

The question isn't "AI or human?" The question is "How does AI make the human parts shine?"

Field Lesson 1: Augmentation Versus Replacement—The Evidence

What AI Reveals

The debate about AI replacing clinicians misses the fundamental insight. Demis Hassabis put it this way in a recent conversation: "If we build artificial general intelligence and compare it to the real mind, we will see what's special and remaining about the human mind—perhaps creativity, perhaps emotions, perhaps consciousness." AI doesn't diminish what makes humans valuable. It illuminates it. But there's an uncomfortable truth alongside this. AI also reveals problems that existed before it arrived. Health care was already treating documentation as a checkbox exercise rather than clinical thinking. Clinicians were already drowning in administrative burden. AI doesn't create these problems; it exposes them by demonstrating how much "clinical work" was actually routine data processing. What remains after automation reveals what should have been protected all along.

What the Evidence Shows

Ambient clinical documentation represents augmentation's most mature example. By January 2025, the category generated $600 million annually, with three major platforms competing: Nuance's DAX Copilot at 33% market share, Abridge at 30% and Ambience Healthcare at 13%. Kaiser Permanente deployed Abridge across 40 hospitals and 600+ medical offices—health care's largest generative AI rollout and Kaiser's fastest technology implementation in over 20 years.

The results prove measurable. A multi-site study published in JAMA Network Open showed burnout dropped from 51.9% to 38.8% after 30 days of ambient AI scribe use.[7] Sutter Health's 100-clinician Abridge evaluation showed decreased time per note, improved satisfaction and reduced cognitive load. Cleveland Clinic's year-long pilot evaluated five ambient products among 250 physicians spanning 80+ specialties before selecting Ambience Healthcare and disseminating AI Scribe to 4,000+ physicians and advanced practice providers by spring 2025.[8] Early reviews confirmed what the data suggested: This actually works.

But these successes illuminate something harder to quantify. Physicians spend one hour documenting for every five hours of patient care—"pyjama time" for the evenings it consumes. Ambient scribes cut documentation by more than 50%, but the real value isn't time saved. It's what clinicians do with it.

They look at patients. They listen. They think. They integrate context. They exercise clinical judgement. They build therapeutic relationships. These activities don't appear on efficiency dashboards, but they're what medicine is actually for.

What AI Cannot Do

Current evidence confirms AI's strengths in pattern recognition, data synthesis and rule-based processing. But four capabilities remain distinctly human, and any augmentation strategy that ignores them will fail.

1. The first is clinical judgement—knowing when standard protocols don't apply, when the textbook answer misses the patient's actual situation and when guidelines conflict and trade-offs must be weighed.

2. The second is patient relationship: building trust, communicating uncertainty, navigating family dynamics, delivering difficult news and understanding what the patient values beyond clinical outcomes.

3. The third is ethical reasoning: balancing beneficence and autonomy, navigating conflicts between patient wishes and medical recommendations, recognising when cultural or religious considerations override clinical optimisation.

4. The fourth is context integration: understanding that the lonely elderly patient might benefit more from a medication requiring daily clinic visits than a more effective drug that isolates them at home or that the single parent working three jobs needs a treatment plan that fits their life rather than the theoretically optimal one.

AI makes all of this possible by handling what machines do well: creating cognitive space for what only humans can provide.

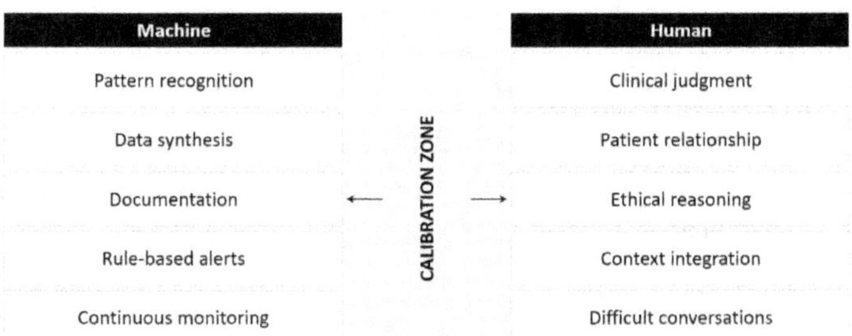

Figure 9. The calibration zone shifts as appropriate trust is built. Neither blind acceptance nor wholesale rejection. AI handles what machines do well; humans retain what only humans can provide.

Field Lesson 2: Trust and Collaboration Calibration

The Over-Trust Problem

Augmentation introduces a paradox: Clinicians must trust AI enough to rely on it but not so much that they defer when their judgement is better. Calibration matters more than capability.

Research on clinical decision support reveals a consistent pattern. When AI provides recommendations, some clinicians accept them without adequate scrutiny, even when clinical judgement suggests otherwise. This isn't laziness; it's cognitive offloading in the context of overwhelming workload and decision fatigue.

The question becomes, "Is over-reliance a technology problem or a systems problem?" The answer is both. AI systems that present recommendations without transparent reasoning encourage blind acceptance. But clinicians who lack cognitive space for genuine thinking—who face patient volumes that preclude deliberation—will defer to any tool that promises to reduce cognitive load. The solution isn't removing AI. It's redesigning work so clinicians have capacity for the thinking that actually matters.

Creating Time for Thinking

Ambient documentation provides one model: Automate the automatable so humans can focus on the irreducibly human. The principle extends beyond documentation. Diagnostic support systems should surface relevant patterns without dictating conclusions. Treatment planning tools should generate options while preserving clinical judgement about which fits this patient's situation. The goal isn't efficiency at the expense of expertise. It's efficiency that enables expertise.

A study of ambient documentation adoption found rates typically range from 20 – 50% when widely available, though one organisation achieved 75 – 80% by emphasising note customisation followed by hands-on training.[9] Massachusetts General Brigham reported that approximately 90% of ambulatory primary care physicians requested access—demand driven by word-of-mouth experience from early adopters who found the technology actually delivered on its promise. The distinction between superusers, variable users and non-users reveals something important: Adoption succeeds when clinicians experience AI as augmentation, not as disruption. When the technology fits workflow rather than forcing workflow to fit technology. When customisation reflects practice patterns rather than imposing standardisation.

Calibrating Trust

Successful implementations frame AI as a collaborative partner, not a replacement. Human-in-the-loop design maintains clinician authority while providing AI support. Transparency about AI limitations builds appropriate scepticism. Training emphasises when to trust AI and when to question it.

But trust calibration requires something deeper: clear accountability frameworks. When AI makes a recommendation and a clinician accepts it, who owns the outcome if it's wrong? Current legal ambiguity creates either paralysis (clinicians second-guess every AI suggestion, defeating the purpose) or abdication (blind acceptance because "the AI said so"). Neither serves patients. Until health care establishes explicit legal clarity about responsibility for AI-assisted decisions, trust calibration will remain incomplete. Chapter 3's liability toolkit provides a starting framework: phased deployment, defined human-in-the-loop thresholds, documentation standards and kill-switch protocols.

Calibration requires three elements working together:

"Transparency" means clinicians need to understand what AI is doing and why; black boxes encourage either blind acceptance or wholesale rejection.

"Feedback loops" mean that when clinicians override AI recommendations, the system should learn, and when AI suggestions prove accurate, clinicians should see evidence. Mutual learning builds calibrated trust.

"Cognitive space" means trust calibration requires thinking; if clinicians lack time to evaluate AI outputs, they'll either accept blindly or ignore entirely.

The best augmentation strategies create time for the deliberation that builds appropriate trust.

Field Lesson 3: Agentic AI—The Next Frontier

From Passive to Active

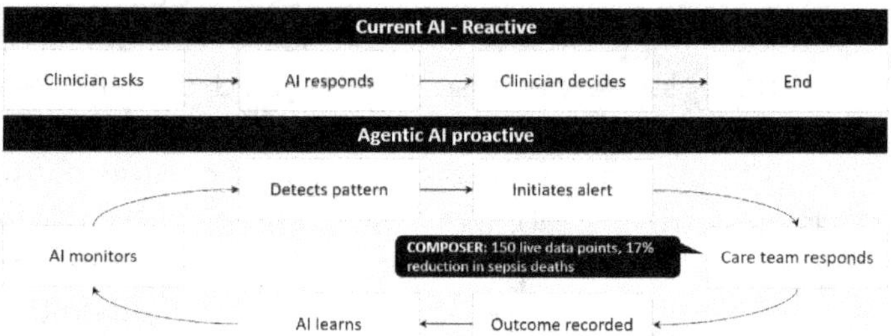

Figure 10. Current AI responds when asked. Agentic AI monitors continuously, detects patterns, initiates alerts and learns from outcomes, as demonstrated by Duke's COMPOSER (17% reduction in sepsis deaths).

Current AI systems are reactive; they respond when prompted. The next generation is agentic; they take initiative, operate autonomously and act to achieve goals with limited oversight. This represents a fundamental shift from tools that assist to agents that act.

Traditional clinical decision support waits for clinicians to query it. Agentic AI monitors continuously, identifies problems and initiates responses autonomously. UC San Diego's COMPOSER system exemplifies this shift; it watches 150 live data points from ED patients, autonomously predicts sepsis onset hours before clinical symptoms appear and alerts the clinical team. A 6,000-case study published in January 2024[10] showed the system cut sepsis deaths by 17%. That's not decision support. That's an autonomous agent acting to achieve a goal—prevent sepsis mortality—by executing a plan: continuous monitoring, early detection, targeted alerting.

Gartner predicts agentic AI usage will surge from less than 1% of enterprise applications in 2024 to 33% by 2028. The global agentic AI market is projected to reach $200 billion by 2034. Health care will be at the forefront of this transformation whether it's ready or not.

What Agentic AI Enables and Where It Struggles

Autonomous clinical decision support that continuously analyses patient data, identifies deterioration and escalates concerns before crises occur. Intelligent care coordination that navigates complex treatment plans across multiple specialties, schedules tests, books follow-up appointments and ensures nothing falls through the cracks. Predictive resource allocation that anticipates ICU needs, operating room utilisation and staffing requirements days in advance. Catalonia's public health service implemented Advanced Learning Medical Assistant (ALMA) to keep 20,000 health care professionals current with constantly changing medical guidelines. The system doesn't wait for clinicians to search; it proactively surfaces relevant updates based on practice patterns and current cases. This is the power of agentic AI: systems that anticipate needs, coordinate across silos and maintain continuity without requiring constant human orchestration.

But there's a domain constraint worth being honest about. Autonomous agents excel in well-defined contexts with clear goals and measurable outcomes. Sepsis has biomarkers and escalation protocols. Care coordination for straightforward cases follows predictable patterns.

But what happens when agentic systems face ambiguity? When clinical guidelines conflict? When patient values override clinical optimisation? When social determinants matter more than medical algorithms? The honest answer is that we don't know yet. Health care contains many domains that aren't well-defined, and that's where agentic AI will struggle.

What Agentic AI Demands

Hassabis himself acknowledges the trade-off: The next stage is agent-based systems, more autonomous. And the risks go up as well. Agentic systems introduce challenges that reactive systems avoid.

1. Infrastructure readiness

   Autonomous agents need resilient, well-integrated systems to act within. They expose infrastructure fragility that human workarounds previously masked. Many platforms actively block agent access because their systems can't handle autonomous operations. If your infrastructure isn't ready, agentic AI will either fail or cause cascading problems, and the platform thinking from Chapter 4 becomes a prerequisite, not an option.

2. Trust and identity

   When an AI agent orders tests, schedules procedures or modifies treatment plans, who is responsible? How do audit trails work? How do clinicians maintain situational awareness when AI acts without prompting?

3. Privacy and security

   Agentic systems access and integrate data across boundaries that human workflows respect through training and social norms. AI agents need explicit permission frameworks, access controls and data governance that match their autonomous capabilities.

4. Governance frameworks

   Reactive AI operates within requests; agentic AI initiates actions. This requires defining what decisions agents can make autonomously, what requires human approval, how to escalate uncertain situations and how to maintain human oversight without creating bottlenecks that defeat the purpose of automation.

The organisations succeeding with agentic AI recognise these challenges early. They build governance before deployment, test infrastructure capacity before scaling and design human-agent collaboration patterns that maintain appropriate oversight without micromanagement.

Field Lesson 4: Engagement Over Approval

Two Models of Human-AI Collaboration

The difference between augmentation and automation lies in feedback loops. Automation eliminates human involvement. Augmentation creates structured dialogue between humans and machines, where both improve through interaction.

Many AI implementations follow an "approval model": AI generates output; humans review and approve. This treats clinicians as quality control—a bottleneck that AI must pass through before proceeding. The better model is engagement: AI and clinicians working together, each contributing what they do best, with ongoing dialogue that improves both.

Consider ambient documentation. The approval model would be AI transcribes and generates notes, clinician reviews and signs. This treats documentation as a pass/fail quality check. The engagement model looks different: AI captures conversation and generates draft note, clinician reviews while the encounter is fresh in memory, corrects errors, adds context AI missed and provides feedback that improves future performance. Over time, the AI learns what this specific clinician considers important, how they structure notes and what details they consistently add. The clinician gets better notes with less effort. The AI gets better at generating notes that match clinical needs. Both improve through dialogue.

Building Learning Loops

Microsoft's journey with DAX Copilot illustrates the importance of feedback. From 2014 to 2023, they struggled with incremental progress, stuck at error rates that prevented automation at scale. The breakthrough came not from better transcription but from structured learning, capturing what clinicians corrected, understanding why recommendations were accepted or rejected and iteratively improving based on real-world clinical judgement. The system doesn't just reduce documentation time. It learns what good documentation looks like for different specialties, different practice patterns and different clinical contexts.

Engagement means clinicians develop new skills: knowing what questions to ask AI, recognising when AI outputs warrant scepticism and understanding how to provide feedback that actually improves performance. This isn't about replacing clinical education; it's expanding it. Just as clinicians learnt to interpret lab values, imaging studies and monitoring data, they're now learning to engage with AI-generated insights, recommendations and analyses. The best implementations treat this as professional development, not just technology training. They teach clinicians how AI works, what its limitations are, when to trust it and how to collaborate effectively. They create cultures where questioning AI is valued, not dismissed as technophobia.

The Feedback Infrastructure

Feedback loops require infrastructure. Systems need to capture when clinicians override recommendations and why. When AI suggestions prove accurate and when they miss. What modifications clinicians consistently make and what that reveals about AI's blind spots. Organisations implementing this well assign responsibility: who reviews feedback patterns, who decides when AI needs retraining and who determines when performance warrants expanding usage versus pulling back. This infrastructure isn't optional for agentic AI; it's essential. Autonomous agents need even stronger feedback mechanisms because they act without prompting. The systems monitoring agent behaviour, detecting drift from intended behaviour and flagging problems before they cascade become critical safety infrastructure.

Framework Close: Augmentation Design Principles

Before designing or deploying any AI system that touches clinical work, the leadership team should be able to answer four questions clearly. If they can't, the implementation will fail in predictable ways.

1. What decisions require human judgement that AI can inform but not replace, and have we made those boundaries explicit in system design, clinical training and governance frameworks rather than leaving it to individual clinicians to figure out?
2. Where can AI free up time for the irreducibly human parts of care, and what will clinicians actually do with that time? If the answer is "see more patients", we've missed the point.
3. How will clinicians engage with AI recommendations—through approval (which treats them as quality control bottlenecks) or through dialogue (which treats them as collaborators who make the AI better)?
4. Is our infrastructure ready for agentic AI? Can our systems handle real-time data integration across silos? Do we have governance frameworks for autonomous decision-making? Are audit trails and accountability mechanisms clear? Can we detect when agents drift from intended behaviour? Do we have kill switches and escalation protocols?

Back to Samantha

Samantha thinks about Dr Hassan's appointment. The ambient documentation worked; the notes appeared faster and more complete than any manual entry could achieve. But what mattered wasn't the notes.

It was Dr Hassan's taking Margaret's hand when she asked about time. The way he created space for fear, for hope, for honesty about uncertainty. The clinical judgement to recognise when protocols matter less than presence. The AI captured the conversation. Dr Hassan provided what the conversation needed.

This is augmentation: technology handling what technology does well so humans can provide what only humans can provide. Not replacement. Not automation. Collaboration that makes both more capable. Samantha also notices something else. Three months in, Dr Hassan's team has developed instincts about when the AI misses context, when generated notes need clinical correction and when suggestions warrant questioning. They've learnt to engage with the technology, not just approve its outputs.

But she also recalls her mother's initial confusion about the recording. Organisations implementing ambient documentation must address patient privacy explicitly. This means clear informed consent before recording begins, transparency about how AI processes conversations and genuine patient choice to opt out without affecting care quality. Some patients appreciate knowing everything is captured accurately. Others feel uncomfortable being recorded. Both preferences deserve respect. Governance structures must ensure recordings are secure, access is audited and retention policies balance clinical utility against privacy protection. The technology enables better documentation, but trust requires transparency about when patients are being observed and how their words become data.

The system is learning too. Fewer corrections each week. Better matching of documentation to practice patterns. Iterative improvement through dialogue. This is the augmentation playbook: clear boundaries between human and machine domains, feedback loops that improve both, engagement over approval, infrastructure that supports autonomous operation safely. And time—precious, scarce, essential time—for clinicians to think, to judge, to care in ways that matter.

Remember the Five Things

These aren't five separate design choices. They're a connected system, and what holds them together is the recognition that augmentation succeeds when technology serves clinical judgement rather than substituting for it.

1. AI reveals the human.

   Not as rhetoric but as operational reality. Once machines handle pattern recognition and documentation, what's left is the work that should have been protected all along. The clinicians spending time with patients instead of screens aren't doing less work. They're doing the work medicine is actually for.

2. Calibration matters more than capability.

   The most accurate AI in the world is dangerous in the hands of clinicians who can't tell when to trust it and when to override it. Transparency, feedback loops and cognitive space—these are the calibration infrastructure. Without them, you get either automation bias or wholesale rejection.

3. Agentic AI changes everything.

   But only for organisations whose infrastructure, governance and accountability frameworks are ready for autonomous systems. The COMPOSER 17% mortality reduction shows what's possible. The platform thinking from Chapter 4 is the prerequisite. Skip the foundations and agentic AI fails or worse, succeeds at the wrong things.

4. Engagement beats approval.

   Dialogue makes both clinicians and AI better, while approval treats clinicians as bottlenecks. The Microsoft DAX Copilot story is the clearest evidence: The breakthrough came from structured learning, not from better transcription. Build the feedback loops and the system improves continuously. Skip them and you're maintaining static technology in a changing clinical environment.

5. Create time for thinking.

   This is the test that matters most. Every augmentation decision should be evaluated against this question: Does this give clinicians more cognitive space for judgement, or does it just compress more work into the same time? If the answer is the latter, you've automated the wrong things.

Chapter 7 addresses the question Dr Hassan's team had to answer first: How do you prepare an entire workforce for this shift? Not just doctors but nurses, administrators, informaticists, the whole ecosystem health care requires. The technology changes fast. People—their skills, their confidence, their understanding of how to work alongside AI—change more slowly. The workforce equation matters as much as the technology equation. Maybe more.

Chapter 7
The Workforce Equation

Preparing People for AI-Enabled Health Care

Key message: Technology changes fast. People change more slowly. The workforce question isn't "Will jobs disappear?" but "How do we help people navigate what's coming?" Focus on the work to be done, not just the roles. New jobs-to-be-done require new roles, and existing roles will transform. This isn't only about preparing for tomorrow. It's about addressing today's crisis: EDs at unsafe ratios, primary care physicians retiring faster than graduates enter practice, nursing vacancies forcing unit closures. The long-term transformation and the current crisis require the same solution: investing in people alongside technology.

If You Read Nothing Else, Remember These Five Things

1. The work transforms before the role does.

   Medical coding won't disappear, but what medical coders do will change fundamentally. Medical secretaries won't vanish, but their work will shift from routine scheduling to exception handling and complex coordination. The role persists; the underlying work evolves. Honest organisations acknowledge that exception handling is harder work than routine processing and adjust compensation accordingly.

2. AI literacy is the new baseline.

   Just as EMR proficiency became non-negotiable, understanding how to engage with AI systems is now foundational across all health care roles. But comprehensive four-hour training programmes don't work; completion rates hover at 20%. What works is micro-learning at the point of need: short modules on specific capabilities, peer support from AI champions and the 12-term vocabulary from Chapter 2 as a foundation.

3. New roles are emerging faster than training programmes can respond.

   Forward deployed clinical engineers (FDEs), clinical informaticists, AI oversight specialists, human-AI workflow designers, algorithmic auditors—these roles didn't exist five years ago. They're critical today. Organisations that develop these capabilities internally, building from people who already understand health care's complexity, outperform those competing for scarce external talent.

4. Where AI leadership sits matters.

   Reporting through clinical informatics versus IT produces different priorities, different outcomes and different organisational cultures around AI adoption. The best models create dual reporting with explicit governance: clinical authority over use case selection, technical authority over infrastructure and a co-chaired governance committee where the perspectives integrate.

5. Sustaining momentum requires visible wins.

   Sustaining momentum requires visible wins because initial enthusiasm fades and the flywheel builds through regular implementation successes that compound over time, not three-year transformation promises.

   Quarterly wins, transparent adoption metrics and feedback loops where early successes compound—this is how you keep the workforce engaged through a multi-year shift.

Opening

The Staff Consultation

Samantha sits in a staff consultation session about the trust's AI strategy. The room feels tense before anyone speaks.

A medical secretary, Janet, 15 years here, raises her hand. "Am I going to lose my job?" Silence. Everyone's thinking it. Janet said it. Samantha knows the honest answer is complicated. Some administrative work will disappear. Scheduling coordination, basic documentation, routine follow-ups—AI handles these increasingly well. But new work is emerging in contexts nobody anticipated. Work demanding human judgement where AI can't reach.

She thinks of her niece Emma, just finishing a health informatics degree, hired before graduation by an AI startup building clinical workflow tools. Emma's role, FDE, didn't exist when Samantha started her career. It combines clinical knowledge, technical capability and embedded operational understanding. Three disciplines that training programmes kept separate now converge in a single role.

She thinks of her colleague Sarah, who left last month. Not because of job loss but because of opportunity. Sarah joined Abridge as a clinical validation specialist. The role requires nursing experience plus understanding of AI system behaviour plus ability to bridge clinical and engineering teams. Sarah's salary doubled.

The workforce isn't just a "change management" problem to solve with better communications. These are real people with mortgages, families and career investments spanning decades. Janet's question deserves a real answer.

Samantha speaks carefully. "Some tasks will change. Some will automate. Let me be honest with you. Transition takes years and requires organisational support. Not everyone will successfully reskill. That's a reality we need to acknowledge. But health care employment is growing 13% through 2032—faster than automation can displace overall. The workforce is bifurcating. Routine work compresses while judgement-intensive work expands dramatically. Care coordinators for complex cases, clinical informaticists, oversight specialists—these roles are growing fast. The question isn't whether yours exists. It's what work that role does and how we help you develop the skills for what's coming. That support is our responsibility, not yours alone."

Janet nods slowly. Not convinced. But listening.

The question isn't "Will jobs disappear?" The question is "How do we help people navigate what's coming?"

Field Lesson 1: The Skills Reality

The Training Gap That Isn't About Computer Literacy

Health care organisations face a challenge: 43% of professionals report that lack of IT expertise delays digital transformation. The training gap isn't about basic computer literacy. It's about understanding how AI systems work, when to trust them, what questions to ask and how to provide feedback that improves performance. Comprehensive training programmes sound good on paper. Four-hour courses covering AI fundamentals, ethics, technical capabilities and clinical applications. Organisations launch them with fanfare. Three months later, completion rates hover around 20%. The content sits in learning management systems, rarely accessed, quickly forgotten.

The problem isn't course quality; it's the delivery model. Time-poor clinicians can't block four hours for training that feels theoretical. They need learning that fits workflow, addresses immediate problems and builds competency through practice.

What Works: Micro-Learning at the Point of Need

The organisations succeeding with AI literacy take a different approach: micro-learning modules at the point of need. Five-minute videos on specific capabilities. Quick-reference guides for common questions. Just-in-time support when clinicians encounter new features.

This connects directly to Chapter 2's 12-term vocabulary. AI literacy doesn't require data science degrees. It requires vocabulary to ask intelligent questions and recognise non-answers. Algorithm. Training data. Validation. Bias. Model drift. Explainability. Twelve terms provide the foundation for productive engagement. Build from there iteratively. Don't front-load comprehensive knowledge. Develop competency through repeated, practical application in clinical context. Northwell Health's approach exemplifies this. Rather than mandated training, they created "AI champions" in each department—clinicians who develop deeper expertise and provide peer support. When colleagues encounter questions, they ask champions first. Learning happens in context, addresses real problems and builds from actual workflow friction rather than hypothetical scenarios.

The Literacy Assessment

Before launching training, assess the current state. Not with surveys asking "How comfortable are you with AI?" Those produce reassuring numbers and zero insight. Use practical scenarios instead. Given this AI recommendation, what questions would you ask before accepting it? "This algorithm was trained on academic medical centre data. What concerns does that raise for community hospital implementation?" "The system flagged this patient as high-risk for readmission. What additional context do you need to act on that alert?"

The answers reveal gaps between current capability and needed competency. Training then targets specific deficits rather than covering everything superficially.

Field Lesson 2: The Change Champion Model

A Different Kind of Leadership

AI implementation requires leadership, but not the traditional kind. Not executives announcing transformation from boardrooms. Not IT directors deploying technology from behind computer screens. The organisations succeeding build change champion networks—clinicians and staff who bridge technical capability, clinical context and frontline reality.

Effective AI champions develop competency across four domains:

1. Technical capability

   Understanding how AI systems work. Not coding them, but grasping training methods, validation approaches, performance metrics and limitation patterns. Enough knowledge to ask intelligent questions and interpret technical responses.

2. Adaptive capacity

   Recognising when workflows need redesign versus when technology needs adjustment, seeing where friction indicates system problems versus change resistance, understanding the difference between bugs and feature limitations.

3. Change leadership

   Building coalitions, addressing concerns without dismissing them, celebrating early wins, sustaining momentum when initial enthusiasm fades. Change leadership isn't about overcoming resistance; it's about creating conditions where adaptation feels possible.

4. AI governance

    Understanding accountability frameworks, privacy implications, equity considerations and regulatory requirements. Knowing when decisions need escalation versus local resolution.

Traditional clinical training doesn't develop these skills. Traditional IT training misses clinical context. The champion model succeeds because it develops all four deliberately.

Phase Zero, Not Pilots

Most organisations talk about "pilots"—small-scale tests before broader rollout. But pilots often design for success in controlled environments rather than scalability in messy reality. They prove technology works but don't answer the question that actually matters: "Can this scale?" Phase Zero thinking designs differently. From day one, ask, "What prevents this from scaling? What workflow dependencies will break at volume? What training gaps will surface when 100 clinicians adopt simultaneously instead of five volunteers?" Phase Zero isn't a pilot. It's deliberate design for scale, tested first in a constrained environment but built with expansion assumptions baked in. The infrastructure, the training, the support model, the feedback mechanisms—all architected for thousands of users from the start, even if initial deployment serves dozens. Tampa General Hospital's work with Palantir Technologies exemplifies this. They didn't pilot sepsis detection; they embedded Palantir engineers in clinical operations from the beginning, building for hospital-wide deployment while learning from initial implementation. The result: 700+ lives saved through Sepsis Hub and infrastructure ready for expansion to other use cases without rebuilding the foundation.

Where AI Leadership Sits

Organisational placement shapes priorities. AI leadership reporting through clinical informatics produces different outcomes than leadership reporting through IT.

Clinical reporting emphasises clinical validation, workflow integration and adoption support. Technology serves clinical goals. Decisions prioritise patient care impact over technical elegance. IT reporting emphasises technical architecture, system integration and infrastructure robustness. Clinical needs filter through technical feasibility. Decisions prioritise scalable solutions over departmental customisation. Both perspectives are needed. Both are valid. The best models create dual reporting with explicit governance: clinical authority over use case selection and validation, technical authority over infrastructure and integration and a governance committee with clinical and technical co-chairs that addresses conflicts through clear decision frameworks. Clinical validation decisions follow the clinical path. Infrastructure decisions follow the technical path. Use case prioritisation requires both perspectives, and the governance committee provides the forum where they integrate.

Cleveland Clinic provides one working model: Their chief clinical transformation officer has authority over use case selection but partners formally with the CIO on implementation. It's not perfect, but it's better than most organisations' ambiguous structures.

Where organisations fail: putting AI leadership in positions without authority over resources, without clinical credibility or without technical depth. Change champions need all three to succeed.

Field Lesson 3: Engaging the Whole Workforce

Janet's Question Deserves a Real Answer

Janet's question, "Am I going to lose my job?", reflects legitimate concern. Dismissing it as resistance to change misses the point. Job security fears are rational when automation eliminates tasks, even if new work emerges. The organisations handling this well don't sugarcoat reality. They acknowledge, yes, some tasks will automate. Documentation will require fewer hours. Scheduling will need less manual coordination. Basic triage will happen through AI systems before human involvement. But they reframe: The role might not change, but the underlying work will. Medical secretaries won't disappear but their work shifts from scheduling to exception handling, from routine documentation to complex care coordination, from transactional tasks to relationship-intensive support.

This requires honesty about something organisations often miss. Exception handling is harder work. When Janet shifts from routine scheduling to managing complex cases that AI can't resolve, her job gets more difficult, not less. It demands different skills, greater judgement and more cognitive load. Organisations must acknowledge this openly and adjust compensation accordingly. If the work increased in complexity, the recognition should too. This isn't semantic wordplay. It's honest recognition that job-to-be-done matters more than job title.

The Historical Parallel

When automobiles replaced horse-drawn carriages, blacksmiths didn't become obsolete; they became automotive mechanics. The role transformed because the underlying work transformed. Similar skills (metalwork, problem-solving, mechanical systems) applied differently. Health care faces an analogous shift. Clinical knowledge remains essential, but application contexts change. The nurse who understands both patient care and AI system behaviour becomes more valuable, not less. The administrative coordinator who excels at exception handling—the cases AI can't resolve—becomes indispensable. The challenge: This transition takes time, requires retraining and demands organisational support. Simply announcing "adapt or leave" fails both people and organisation.

Building Internal Pipelines

Northwell Health's reskilling framework provides a model. One nurse learns data analysis and information management, transitioning toward a clinical informaticist role. Another pursues training for management positions, drawing on expertise in operational leadership. A third seeks mentorship preparing for patient advocacy work. Career mobility. Organisational agility. The workforce develops capability that allows adaptation, the organisation builds internal pipelines rather than depending on external talent markets and individuals see pathways forward that honour their invested experience while acknowledging changed reality.

Global Data found 47% of cybersecurity jobs going unfilled. AI roles show similar gaps— a 50% hiring shortfall. Health care can't compete in external markets for technical talent. But it can develop talent internally from people who already understand health care's complexity. The same dual-win principle from Chapter 3 applies: External partnerships and consultants accelerate capability building, but the goal is organisational muscle, not permanent dependence.

Sustaining Momentum

Initial enthusiasm is easy. Launch events, executive speeches, early adopter excitement—organisations generate momentum quickly. Sustaining it requires something harder: visible quarterly wins that compound over time.

The flywheel metaphor captures this. Early rotation resists. It's slow, hard work to get moving. But each successful implementation makes the next easier. Adoption builds trust. Trust enables data sharing. Better data improves AI performance. Better AI increases adoption. Round again. Faster.

Organisations that understand this plan for it. They celebrate regular wins publicly. They share adoption metrics transparently. They create feedback loops where early successes compound rather than getting lost in the next transformation initiative. Three years of transformation promises don't motivate. Regular implementation wins building toward transformation do.

Field Lesson 4: Role Evolution Patterns

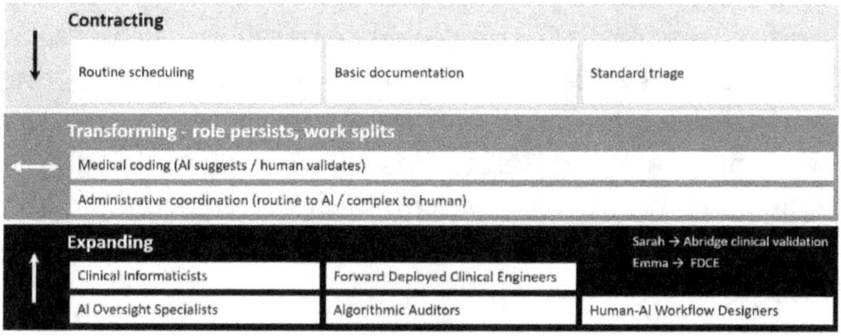

Figure 11. Health care AI roles are contracting (routine tasks automated), transforming (work splits between AI and human) or expanding (new roles: clinical informaticists, FDCEs, AI oversight specialists).

The Forward Deployed Clinical Engineer

New roles are emerging faster than training programmes adapt. Understanding these patterns helps organisations anticipate needs rather than scrambling to fill gaps reactively.

Palantir Technologies pioneered Forward Deployed Engineers—technical professionals embedded in client operations, combining software engineering with domain expertise and implementation ownership. Health care is adapting this model: FDEs who combine clinical knowledge, technical capability and operational integration. Health care AI startups are leading adoption. Bayesian Health, Abridge, Trellis AI are all hiring FDE-style roles. These positions didn't exist in traditional health care organisational charts.

They don't fit neat boxes in HR systems. But they're becoming critical for successful AI implementation.

What they do: work embedded in clinical operations, understand both technical AI capabilities and clinical workflow realities, translate between engineering and clinical teams, own implementation from pilot through scale and iterate based on frontline feedback. This isn't consulting. It's embedded partnership. It's not temporary deployment. It's sustained operational integration.

The New Roles Crystallising

Beyond FDEs, several new roles are taking shape.

Clinical informaticists are physician-level professionals specialising in health care technology. They ensure AI tools meet clinical needs and safety standards. Demand is growing as hospitals integrate AI solutions. These roles command premium salaries in the US market ($150K – $350K+) because they bridge clinical expertise with technology oversight. AI oversight specialists monitor algorithm performance, detect model drift, validate outputs against clinical ground truth and manage governance frameworks—the quality assurance layer for autonomous systems.

Human-AI workflow designers map how humans and AI systems share work optimally designing interfaces, feedback mechanisms and collaboration patterns that enable augmentation rather than replacement. Algorithmic auditors assess AI systems for bias, fairness, performance disparities across populations and compliance with emerging regulations; as regulatory frameworks mature, these roles will become mandatory for health care AI deployment.

AI prompt engineers optimise how clinicians interact with AI systems by crafting queries, designing interfaces and validating outputs.

The Roles Transforming

Some roles don't emerge; they evolve.

Administrative functions reduce in volume but increase in complexity: less time on routine tasks, more time on exception handling, relationship management and complex coordination that AI can't resolve.

Medical coding transforms from manual assignment to validation and oversight. AI suggests codes; humans verify accuracy, handle edge cases and manage appeals when payer systems disagree.

Clinical roles gain AI augmentation across specialties. Radiologists interpret alongside AI detection systems, pathologists review with AI-assisted screening and emergency physicians triage with predictive analytics. The core clinical work persists, now aided by AI partners.

The pattern: Roles requiring pure pattern recognition and rule-based processing face compression. Roles requiring judgement, context integration and human interaction expand. The middle ground—roles combining routine and complex work—splits into components: AI handles routine and humans handle complex.

Framework Close: Workforce Readiness

Workforce transformation requires honest assessment across four dimensions. The leadership team should be able to answer four questions clearly before committing to any AI strategy at scale.

Can our workforce demonstrate practical AI literacy measured through scenario-based competency, not comfort surveys, and do we have a development pathway for those who can't yet?

Where does AI leadership sit in our organisation, and does that placement give it authority over both clinical use case selection and technical infrastructure decisions?

Are we mapping role evolution by jobs-to-be-done rather than defending job titles? And have we adjusted compensation to reflect that exception handling is harder work, not easier?

Are we sustaining momentum through visible quarterly wins and transparent adoption metrics, or are we relying on launch announcements and three-year transformation promises that nobody believes?

Back to Samantha

Two months after Janet's question, Samantha runs into her in the corridor. Janet has just finished a session with the trust's first AI champion, a senior nurse who's been trained to support colleagues through the transition.

"It's not what I expected," Janet says. "I thought I'd be replaced. But the AI champion showed me something. The system can handle the routine bookings now. Mostly. But when something goes wrong, when a patient needs three appointments coordinated across two specialties and a community team, when the family situation is complicated, when the social services referral gets stuck, that's still me. And honestly, it's harder work. The straightforward stuff was easier."

"How are you finding it?"

Janet thinks. "I'm tired. But I feel more useful, somehow. Like I'm doing the work that actually matters. The AI handles the things I used to dread—the endless rebooking, the simple confirmations. I handle the things only I can handle."

She pauses. "I've enrolled in the trust's reskilling programme. Care coordination for complex cases. They're paying for it. I don't know if I'll be brilliant at it. But I know I won't be replaced by software next year either." Samantha thinks about the difference between Janet's first question, "Am I going to lose my job?" and where she is now. The fear hasn't gone. The transition is real. But Janet has something she didn't have at the consultation session: a path forward that honours her experience while acknowledging the changed reality.

That, Samantha realises, is what workforce transformation actually looks like. Not announcements. Not slogans. Specific support for specific people navigating specific changes. The flywheel of trust building one conversation at a time.

She thinks of her niece Emma, the FDE. She thinks of her colleague Sarah, now at Abridge. She thinks of Janet, learning complex care coordination. Three different people. Three different roles. All shaped by the same shift.

The workforce equation isn't about predicting which jobs survive. It's about building organisations where people have the support—and the honesty—to navigate transformation that's already underway.

Remember the Five Things

These aren't five separate workforce initiatives. They're a connected system, and the connection is the recognition that people, not technology, determine whether transformation succeeds.

1. The work transforms before the role does.

   This is why honest organisations distinguish jobs-to-be-done from job titles and adjust compensation when complexity increases. Janet doing exception handling for complex care coordination is doing harder work than Janet booking routine appointments. The honest response isn't "Your job is safe." It's "Your job is changing, and we're investing in you to navigate that change."

2. AI literacy is the new baseline.

   But it's built through micro-learning at the point of need rather than four-hour theoretical courses. Twelve terms from Chapter 2 plus peer support from AI champions plus practical scenarios beats any comprehensive curriculum. Build from clinical context outward, not from theoretical foundations inward.

3. New roles are emerging faster than training programmes.

   FDEs, clinical informaticists, AI oversight specialists, algorithmic auditors. The organisations winning here don't compete for scarce external talent. They build internally from people who already understand health care's complexity. The same dual-win principle from Chapter 3 applies: External partners accelerate, but the goal is organisational muscle.

4. Where AI leadership sits matters.

   Clinical reporting and IT reporting produce different outcomes, and neither alone is sufficient. The best models create dual reporting with explicit governance—clinical authority over use case selection, technical authority over infrastructure, co-chaired governance committees where the perspectives integrate. Ambiguity here is where transformation stalls.

5. Sustaining momentum requires visible wins.

   Initial enthusiasm fades and the flywheel only builds through compounding successes. Quarterly wins, transparent adoption metrics, public celebration of early adopters, feedback loops where early successes inform later deployments—this is how you keep workforce engagement through a multi-year shift. Three-year transformation promises don't motivate. Regular implementation wins do.

Part II ends here. We've moved from seeing clearly (Chapters 1 – 3) through building wisely—the operating system, the ontology layer, the augmentation playbook and now the workforce equation. Foundations are in place. Platforms are built. Ontologies create understanding. AI augments clinicians without replacing them. People are being supported through transition.

But a question hangs over all of it. The board member asks it directly, "What evidence do we have that any of this is actually worth it? How do we measure value? How do we know AI is improving outcomes and not just adding costs?" Part III tackles the hardest questions in the book: proving value when the evidence base is still being built, designing governance that enables rather than paralyses and preparing for capabilities—agentic systems, foundation models, scientific AI—that are arriving faster than most organisations are ready for.

Chapter 8 starts with the value question. It's the question Samantha has been carrying since Chapter 3, when £4.7 million had been spent on seven AI tools and nobody could say whether patients were better off. By the end of Chapter 8, she'll have a framework for answering it honestly, not optimistically, not pessimistically but in a way that lets leadership teams make informed decisions about what to scale, what to pause and what to retire.

PART III: LEADING FORWARD

Chapter 8
The Value Question

Honest Assessment in a World of Inflated Promises

Key message: The question isn't "What's the ROI?" but "What can we honestly claim and what are we still learning?" Organisations that distinguish between outputs they can measure now, outcomes they believe will emerge and learning they are still accumulating make better investment decisions than those accepting vendor business cases uncritically.

If You Read Nothing Else, Remember These Five Things

1. The pilots-to-scale gap is where most health care AI initiatives die.

   Only a small fraction of implementations demonstrate clear financial ROI, not because AI lacks value but because scaling requires changing operating models, not just deploying technology. Organisations stuck in what practitioners call "pilot purgatory" treat AI like science experiments with no accountability. Those achieving sustainable value treat each deployment like a formal project: specific outcome targets, clear accountability, rigorous measurement.

2. Distinguish outputs from outcomes from learning and track all three separately.

   Outputs are what you can measure in 90 days: time savings, efficiency metrics, usage statistics. Outcomes are what you believe will emerge over 12 to 24 months: better patient results, reduced readmissions, improved safety. Learning is what you are still discovering: optimal human-AI collaboration patterns, equity implications, long-term sustainability. Conflating these three categories is how organisations end up governing by hope.

3. Concrete metrics exist when organisations invest in measuring them.

   Kaiser Permanente documented 15,791 physician hours saved through ambient documentation. CommonSpirit Health submitted over 61,000 care gap closure orders in fiscal 2025—a fivefold increase on the prior year—by automating cancer screening guideline adherence. These are not pilot metrics. They are operational results from systems deployed at scale, measured rigorously because someone decided measurement mattered from day one.

4. Leader-led adoption drives results more than technology capability.

   Visa's breakthrough in agentic AI came only after putting their top 300 leaders through hands-on training with the tools they were being asked to fund and govern. CommonSpirit launched an AI Learning Academy in 2025, with over 5,000 course registrations and 1,400 employees upskilled. Technology deployed without leadership understanding produces expensive shelf-ware. Understanding is not a prerequisite for approving a budget line; it is a prerequisite for realising value from it.

5. Define stopping criteria before you start.

   "What would make us stop this investment?" is the question that separates disciplined investing from gambling. Organisations that cannot answer it specifically are not ready to invest. Value documentation that survives scrutiny includes explicit confidence levels for different claims and clear criteria for when to scale, pivot or stop.

Opening

The Board Paper

Samantha stares at the document on her screen, cursor blinking at the end of an unfinished sentence she cannot bring herself to complete.

The chief digital officer (CDO) has asked her to contribute a section on AI investment priorities. She has reviewed the business cases—impressive ROI projections, efficiency gains, cost savings rendered in precise decimals. The slides are beautiful. The numbers are confident. The confidence is, she thinks, the problem.

She asks a simple question in the planning meeting: "Which of these has evidence of improving patient outcomes? Not efficiency. Outcomes."

The room goes quiet. The CFO mentions "strategic value". The CDO talks about "competitive positioning". The chief medical information officer (CMIO) references "emerging literature". Nobody answers her question.

Samantha thinks of her mother. Margaret's cardiologist uses an AI-powered early warning system. It flagged a potential deterioration last month that turned out to be nothing—a false positive that generated an unnecessary hospital visit, additional tests and considerable anxiety for a 74-year-old woman already managing two chronic conditions. The system probably prevents some genuine deteriorations. But how would anyone know? The trust celebrates its sensitivity without mentioning its specificity.

She opens a new section of the document and begins typing, "What we can prove, what we believe and what we don't yet know."

It is the most honest thing in the paper. It will probably be the section most likely to be edited out.

But Samantha has learnt something over two decades in health care. The questions you are not supposed to ask are usually the ones that matter most. And right now, the question nobody wants to answer is whether these investments are actually helping patients or just generating impressive presentations.

Field Lesson 1: The Pilots-to-Scale Problem

Health care organisations love pilots. They are safe and contained and produce encouraging metrics that justify continued investment. The problem is that the vast majority of AI initiatives fail to deliver expected outcomes, and the failure point is almost always the same: the gap between a successful pilot and operational scale.

The pattern repeats across systems. AI gets approached as a technology initiative rather than strategic transformation. Impressive tools get deployed and fail to move meaningful operational metrics. Pilots succeed in controlled environments and struggle when exposed to the full complexity of clinical reality. Technical teams build sophisticated models that clinicians will not use. Compliance becomes an afterthought rather than foundational design.

The root cause is consistent: Organisations focus on what AI can do rather than what problem must be solved and how it will be measured. That distinction sounds simple. It is not. It requires discipline to reject the vendor demonstration that dazzles but cannot specify its outcome metrics, to resist the clinical champion whose enthusiasm exceeds their evidence and to insist on accountability before signing a purchase order.

Other industries have worked this out. At Davos 2026, Saudi Aramco presented 500 AI use cases generating verified value in the billions, not through algorithmic sophistication but through treating each deployment like a formal project with specific profit and loss targets and third-party verification. The key was not the algorithm. It was the accountability structure built around it.

Health care rarely operates this way. A significant proportion of hospitals have not adopted AI at scale, and those that have often remain in what practitioners call "pilot purgatory"— impressive demonstrations that never reach the operational impact they were funded to deliver. The maturity gap is not primarily technical. Scaling requires changing operating models, and that is organisational transformation, the kind most health care leaders have not been trained to execute.

The leading organisations are developing what amounts to a two-speed strategy: fixing fragmented processes and building data foundations while simultaneously running disciplined pilots designed for scale from the start (i.e. Phase 0s). That discipline is not glamorous. It requires saying no to pilots that cannot articulate their success criteria. It requires asking, before any investment is approved, "Are we running a science experiment with no accountability or a formal project with outcome targets and rigorous measurement?"

Field Lesson 2: What Health Care AI Can Actually Measure

The honest admission is that only a small fraction of health care AI implementations demonstrate clear financial ROI. That statistic misleads if taken at face value. The problem is not that AI lacks value; it is that measuring value is genuinely complex, and most organisations have not invested in the measurement infrastructure required.

Where organisations have invested in measurement, the results are striking.

Kaiser Permanente documented 15,791 physician hours saved through ambient documentation. That is roughly seven working years of clinical time returned to patient care. It is not a projection; it is operational data from deployed systems.

CommonSpirit Health, one of the largest non-profit health systems in the United States, deployed an AI-powered care gap closure system across their network. In fiscal 2025, they submitted over 61,000 care gap closure orders—a fivefold increase on the prior year—by automating the complex process of adhering to cancer screening guidelines for breast, colorectal and lung cancer. The system pulls risk factors from electronic health records, calculates personalised screening timelines and recommends appropriate orders to clinicians. The improvement is not a modelled projection. It is a counted difference in clinical actions taken. Cleveland Clinic's autonomous coding system processes large volumes of clinical documents in under two seconds per document. Mount Sinai's emergency department flow optimisation delivered measurable reductions in waiting times and improved bed utilisation. These are operational results, not pilot metrics.

The pattern across these examples is consistent: They measure what matters for their specific context, they track it rigorously and they treat measurement as part of the deployment from day one, not an afterthought appended at the review stage.

What most organisations do not measure is the downstream effect. Does reduced documentation time actually translate to more patient-facing time, or do clinicians simply see more patients in the same hours? Does reduced administrative burden reduce burnout and improve retention? Does better documentation quality affect care coordination and, ultimately, outcomes? These questions require longer time horizons and more sophisticated measurement than most organisations have implemented. The honest approach is to track outputs in 90 days, hypothesise outcomes over 12 to 24 months and document what you are learning continuously rather than waiting until the end of a deployment cycle to discover that nobody captured the data needed to evaluate it.

Field Lesson 3: Outputs, Outcomes and Learning

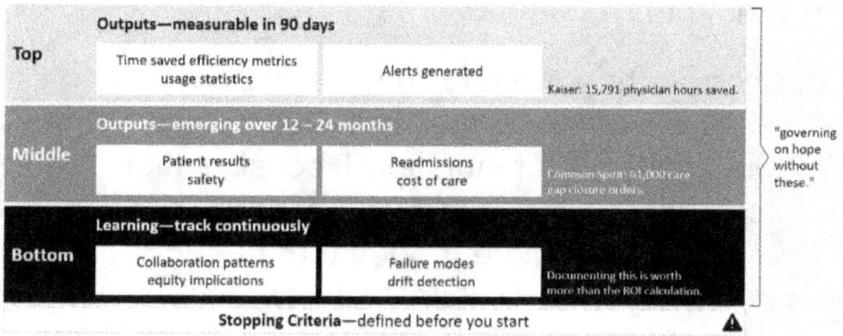

Figure 12. Outputs are measurable in 90 days. Outcomes emerge over 12 to 24 months. Learning must be tracked continuously. Stopping criteria must be defined before you start or you are governing on hope.

The most common mistake in health care AI value assessment is conflating outputs with outcomes. They are not the same thing, and treating them as though they are produces investments that look successful on the dashboard and fail the patient.

Outputs are what can be measured in 90 days. Time saved. Efficiency gains. Usage statistics. Claims processed. Alerts generated. These are operational measures that demonstrate a system is functioning as designed. They are necessary, but they are not the reason anyone invested. Outcomes are what organisations believe will emerge over longer time horizons. Better patient results. Reduced readmissions. Improved safety. Lower total cost of care. These are the reasons investments are made. They require longer measurement windows and more complex attribution, because clinical outcomes are affected by many variables simultaneously and AI is rarely the only thing that changed.

Learning is the category that almost nobody tracks, and it is often where the most valuable insights sit. Optimal patterns of human-AI collaboration. Equity implications across different patient populations. Edge cases and failure modes that did not appear in testing. Long-term sustainability as clinical practice evolves. These insights do not fit neatly into a business case, which is precisely why they get omitted. Omitting them means organisations repeat the same mistakes across successive deployments.

The practical framework follows logically from this structure. Separate your claims by type, and be explicit about what you are measuring directly versus inferring indirectly. Document your assumptions: What has to be true for projected outcomes to materialise? What adoption rates are you assuming? What workflow changes are required? Define stopping criteria before you start. Not "if it fails", which is too vague, but specific metrics at specific thresholds that would trigger a decision to pivot or stop. And track the journey, not just the destination. Document what you expected, what you found and what you changed as a result. That learning documentation is often more valuable than the final ROI calculation. It is what builds organisational capability for future deployments rather than starting from scratch each time. Organisations that cannot distinguish outputs from outcomes from learning are governing on hope. The ones that can are building something that compounds.

Field Lesson 4: Building Value Documentation That Survives Scrutiny

The most sophisticated AI deployment in the world fails if leadership does not understand it. This is not about technical literacy. It is about decision-making capability—the ability to ask the right questions, recognise when something is going off track and distinguish vendor hype from realistic capability.

Visa's experience is instructive. Their breakthrough in agentic AI came only after putting their top 300 leaders through hands-on experience with the technology they were being asked to fund and govern. Not presentations about AI. Not vendor demonstrations. Actual engagement with the tools. That experiential understanding transformed how leadership evaluated proposals, asked questions and made decisions. They could no longer be told what AI could do. They knew.

CommonSpirit Health took a similar approach at scale. Their AI Learning Academy offered both long-form courses and shorter modules, generating over 5,000 course registrations and upskilling more than 1,400 employees within months of launch. That investment in understanding had tangible effects on adoption speed and on the quality of AI use across clinical and operational teams. The training was not compliance. It was capability.

Value documentation that survives scrutiny shares several characteristics. It acknowledges uncertainty explicitly, because different claims carry different confidence levels and pretending otherwise destroys credibility when the scrutiny arrives. High confidence: “We reduced documentation time by 12 minutes per encounter, measured against time-stamped system data.” Medium confidence: “We believe this time saving is being redirected to patient care, based on clinician surveys.” Low confidence: “We expect this will improve patient outcomes over time, though we do not yet have data to demonstrate it.” Each of these is a legitimate claim. Only one of them belongs in a business case headline.

Value documentation also defines stopping criteria before deployment begins. Not aspirationally, specifically. “If clinician adoption remains below 40% after six months of supported implementation, we will review the deployment model.” “If measured time savings fall below eight minutes per encounter, we will reassess the use case.” “If patient complaints increase by more than 10%, we will pause and investigate.” These are the kinds of statements that distinguish organisations investing from organisations gambling. Finally, value documentation treats AI deployments with the same operational discipline applied to capital investment. Phased implementation with clear milestones. Accountability for results at each phase. Third-party verification where the stakes justify it. The rigour that finance applies to a major equipment purchase should be applied to AI deployments, yet in most organisations, it is not.

Framework Close: Honest Value Assessment

Before your next AI investment decision, work through these questions with your leadership team:

What outputs can you measure in 90 days that indicate trajectory? Be specific: which metrics, measured how, against what target thresholds?

What outcomes do you believe will emerge, and when will you know? Separate hypothesis from evidence. Define the time horizon and measurement approach for each claimed outcome, and be explicit about the confidence level you assign to each.

What are you still learning, and how are you documenting that learning? This category is where the most valuable organisational insights accumulate. Do not treat it as optional.

What would make you stop this investment? If you cannot answer this specifically, you are not ready to invest.

Are you treating this as a formal project with outcome targets and accountability or as a science experiment where success is defined after the fact?

The organisations achieving sustainable AI value approach these questions with the same rigour they apply to capital investments. Those stuck in pilot purgatory approach them with good intentions and insufficient discipline.

Back to Samantha

What the CFO Said

Two weeks later, Samantha's section survives the editing process—mostly.

It is the CFO, surprisingly, who champions it. "This is the first honest assessment I've seen in three years of AI proposals," she says in the executive meeting. "I'm tired of approving investments I cannot evaluate."

The board paper now includes a framework borrowed from Samantha's categories. What We Can Prove, with data. What We Believe, with rationale. What We're Learning, with a timeline for review. Each investment proposal must populate all three sections. More importantly, the framework requires stopping criteria. For the first time, the trust is explicitly documenting what would make them discontinue an AI investment, not as pessimism but as discipline. Samantha thinks of her mother again. Margaret's early warning system generated another alert last week—this one legitimate, catching a medication interaction the pharmacy system had missed. The system's value is not zero. But it is also not what the vendor claimed in the sales presentation.

The truth, as usual, is complicated. Complicated truths require honest frameworks to navigate. Samantha is beginning to build one.

Remember the Five Things

These are not five separate evaluation criteria. They form a measurement discipline that compounds over time, and without all five, the others fail.

1. The pilots-to-scale gap is where most health care AI initiatives die.

   The discipline that bridges that gap is treating deployments as formal projects with accountability built in from the start, not as experiments to be evaluated after the fact.

2. Distinguish outputs from outcomes from learning.

   Ninety-day outputs tell you the system is working. Twelve-to-24-month outcomes tell you whether it is working for the reasons you invested. Learning, tracked continuously, tells you what to do differently next time.

3. Concrete metrics exist when organisations invest in measuring them.

   The examples in this chapter—Kaiser Permanente, CommonSpirit, Mount Sinai—are not outliers. They are what rigorous measurement produces. The absence of good metrics is a measurement failure, not an AI failure.

4. Leader-led adoption drives results.

   Understanding is not a nice-to-have. It is the prerequisite for asking the questions that keep AI deployments honest. Visa and CommonSpirit proved this at scale. The investment in leadership capability pays back in every subsequent governance conversation.

5. Define stopping criteria before you start.

   This is the test of whether an organisation is investing or gambling. The value framework built in this chapter—outputs, outcomes, learning, stopping criteria—is only as strong as the discipline applied to all five elements together. Governance (Chapter 9) is where that discipline gets institutionalised.

Chapter 9 explores how to build the architecture of trust that makes AI adoption sustainable, not just for individual investments but for the long-term relationship between your organisation, your clinicians and the patients who depend on both.

Chapter 9
Architecture of Trust

Building Governance That Enables Responsible Innovation

Key message: Trust is infrastructure. Organisations that build it systematically will lead; those that treat it as an afterthought will face adoption barriers that no technology can overcome. In a world where regulatory frameworks are diverging globally and public trust in institutions is at historic lows, governance is not constraint; it is competitive advantage.

If You Read Nothing Else, Remember These Five Things

1. The global regulatory landscape is fragmenting, not converging, and waiting for clarity is a strategy that does not exist.

   The EU AI Act classifies AI-enabled medical devices as high-risk systems, with compliance requirements phasing in through 2027. The US continues a sector-specific, guidance-driven approach with over 1,000 AI-enabled medical devices now authorised by the FDA. China targets 70% AI diffusion by 2027 through a deploy-and-refine philosophy. There is no single framework to align with. Organisations must build adaptive governance that navigates complexity, not governance that waits for consensus.

EU	US	China
• Comprehensive legislation • Phased timeline 2025 – 2027 • High-risk classification for medical AI	• Sector-specific guidance • 1,000+ FDA-authorized • No overarching federal law	• Deploy-and-refine philosophy • 70% AI diffusion target by 2027 • National competitiveness priority

Result: No single framework. Build adaptive governance.

Figure 13. EU: comprehensive legislation, high-risk classification. US: sector specific, 1,000+ FDA-authorised devices. China: deploy and refine, 70% diffusion target by 2027. Result: build adaptive governance.

2. Trust is built through transparency, not opacity.

   Estonia's national health data system lets citizens see exactly who accessed their records and why. That radical transparency paradoxically increased public trust and willingness to share data. The question is not "Is the data secure?" It is "Can patients understand and verify how their data is being used?" These are different questions, and only one of them builds social licence.

3. AI literacy is now a compliance requirement, not a cultural aspiration.

   As of February 2025, the EU AI Act requires that staff dealing with AI systems possess a "sufficient level of AI literacy". This is a legal obligation. Organisations without thorough AI training programmes are already non-compliant with the most comprehensive regulatory framework in existence.

4. Agentic AI requires governance frameworks that most organisations have not yet built.

   When AI systems move from generating recommendations to taking action—booking appointments, ordering tests, coordinating care—the governance question changes fundamentally. Where should AI suggest and wait? Where does it require human approval? Where can it act autonomously within defined guardrails? Most organisations have not answered these questions. They will need to before they deploy systems that cannot be easily recalled.

5. Take the long view seriously, not as philosophical indulgence but as strategic discipline.

   Technological revolutions historically take generations to reach stable states. The Industrial Revolution caused enormous disruption before societies developed the institutions to manage it responsibly. AI is moving faster. The governance infrastructure built now will shape outcomes for decades. Organisations that treat governance as a compliance exercise will be repeatedly surprised. Those that treat it as strategic infrastructure will be ready.

Opening

The Patient Portal

Samantha sits beside her mother at the kitchen table, helping Margaret log in to view her latest test results.

"Who else can see this?" Margaret asks, peering at the screen with the careful attention she gives to anything involving her health.

Samantha opens her mouth to answer, then stops. She works in health care. She should know. But the honest answer is that she does not.

The consent forms Margaret signed are impenetrable —pages of legal language that even Samantha, with two decades in the industry, struggles to parse. The data-sharing agreements are buried in policy documents that reference other policy documents in an endless chain of institutional opacity. And the AI systems now processing her mother's data? They operate under governance frameworks that Samantha, as an operations director, does not fully understand. "I'm not actually sure," Samantha admits. "The trust has data governance policies, but..." Margaret looks at her daughter with the patient expression of someone who has learnt to accept institutional vagueness as a condition of receiving health care. “Well, I suppose they know what they're doing.” Do they? Samantha wonders. If she cannot explain it to her mother, a retired teacher who spent 40 years helping students understand complex ideas, how can patients possibly give informed consent? Trust is not just about security. It is about understanding. And right now, nobody fully understands.

Later that evening, she reads about Estonia's approach to health data governance. Citizens can see exactly who accessed their records and why. They receive notifications when their data is viewed. The radical transparency paradoxically increased public trust and willingness to share data.

She bookmarks the article. Maybe there is a better way.

Field Lesson 1: The Global Regulatory Landscape

The regulatory environment for health care AI is not converging toward global standards. It is actively fragmenting, creating a complex patchwork that multinational organisations must navigate and smaller organisations cannot afford to ignore.

The European Union has produced the world’s most comprehensive attempt to regulate AI. The EU AI Act classifies AI used in medical devices as high-risk, requiring stringent compliance measures that phase in across a structured timeline. February 2025 brought AI literacy requirements and enforcement of prohibited AI practices. August 2025 brought rules for general-purpose AI models. August 2026 brings most provisions for high-risk AI systems, and August 2027 brings full compliance requirements for AI-enabled medical devices. Organisations must implement quality management systems, conduct conformity assessments, report serious incidents to Market Surveillance Authorities within 15 days and ensure human oversight of AI-enabled clinical tools. The Act intersects with existing Medical Device Regulation (MDR) in ways that regulatory analysts describe as creating genuine "regulatory overlap", and industry bodies have warned that parallel frameworks could complicate compliance for smaller providers.

The United States has taken a fundamentally different approach. Rather than comprehensive legislation, the FDA has evolved its guidance through iterative policy development. The agency has authorised more than 1,000 AI-enabled medical devices, with 2024 setting a record for annual authorisations. January 2025 brought comprehensive draft guidance on AI-enabled device software lifecycle management. But there is no overarching federal AI law. Regulation happens through executive orders, agency guidance and a growing patchwork of state-level initiatives with hundreds of separate AI bills introduced across state legislatures in recent years. This creates both opportunity and risk. Organisations can move faster than under EU-style regulation. They also face uncertainty about future requirements and inconsistency across jurisdictions. China represents the third major regulatory philosophy: aggressive deployment with adaptive regulation. The government has set targets for 70% AI diffusion by 2027, rising to 90% by 2030. The approach prioritises national competitiveness over precautionary regulation. For international organisations, this creates a complex calculation—operating in China requires compliance with evolving domestic requirements while China's deploy-and-refine philosophy generates real-world evidence that may not be available elsewhere.

The practical reality is that there is no single framework to align with. Organisations operating internationally must navigate complexity rather than waiting for clarity that will not arrive on a useful timescale. This requires governance flexible enough to accommodate multiple regulatory environments, explicit tracking of developments across relevant jurisdictions and compliance strategies built from the most stringent requirements while retaining adaptability. Regulatory compliance handled as a checkbox exercise will be repeatedly disrupted as requirements evolve. Governance built as adaptive infrastructure will find regulation becoming a source of credibility, demonstrating trustworthiness in a market where trust is increasingly scarce.

Field Lesson 2: International Models and the Question of What Travels

At Davos 2026, Demis Hassabis proposed what he called a "CERN for AI"—an international institution modelled on the European Organisation for Nuclear Research, where scientists from competing nations collaborate on fundamental research, sharing knowledge while maintaining their respective national programmes.

The proposal matters for health care because AI in medicine is fundamentally international. Diseases do not respect borders. Research crosses jurisdictions. AI models trained in one country are deployed in others, often without adequate adaptation to local contexts. Yet there is currently no international framework for health care AI governance. The World Health Organisation has published regulatory considerations emphasising transparency, risk management and continuous monitoring, but these remain guidance, not binding framework, and the gap between guidance and implementation is where most harm occurs.

National models offer lessons, even where direct replication is impossible. Estonia built national infrastructure enabling innovation while maintaining security, with near-universal digital prescriptions and a system that lets patients see who accessed their records and why. Singapore implemented a national patient identifier with mandated interoperability—a technical achievement that smaller, more centralised health systems can accomplish more readily than federated systems like the US or UK. The UAE and Dubai are positioning as AI validation hubs, developing regional frameworks for cross-border health data and trusted research environments that offer organisations operating in the Gulf a governance environment that balances innovation with accountability.

The critical question is not which national model to copy; none of them transfer wholesale. It is what principles travel, even when specific implementations cannot. Several patterns emerge consistently from the cases that have succeeded. Transparency builds trust. When patients can verify who accessed their records and why, they feel more in control and are more willing to share data, even if they rarely exercise that verification in practice. Interoperability enables innovation—the integration work that organisations resist is precisely what makes AI applications possible at scale. And governance frameworks can be adapted across contexts even when technical implementations cannot. The underlying logic of Estonia's transparency feature or Singapore's interoperability mandate is portable in ways that their specific architectures are not.

For health care leaders, the question is whether governance is being built to work across the jurisdictions you operate in or whether you are creating siloed approaches that will require expensive harmonisation once the regulatory landscape clarifies.

Field Lesson 3: Trust as Infrastructure—Building Social Licence

Public trust in technology is at historic lows. Public trust in government institutions is at historic lows. Public trust in health care, while higher than most other sectors, has declined meaningfully since the pandemic. This is the environment in which organisations are asking patients to share their data with AI systems they do not understand, governed by frameworks they cannot access, for benefits they cannot verify.

Social licence is the implicit permission that societies grant to institutions to operate. It is distinct from legal compliance. An organisation can be fully compliant with every applicable regulation while lacking social licence, and when that gap opens, adoption stalls, resistance mounts and beneficial technologies fail to reach the patients they were designed to help.

The Estonia model demonstrates how transparency mechanisms can close this gap. Patients can see exactly who accessed their health records and why. The audit trail is visible to the individual, not just the institution. This seems risky to organisations accustomed to operating behind institutional opacity. Surely patients will complain about every access? The Estonian experience suggests the opposite. Transparency reduces complaints because patients feel respected. Institutions become more careful when they know their access is visible. The perception of oversight, even rarely exercised, changes behaviour on both sides of the relationship.

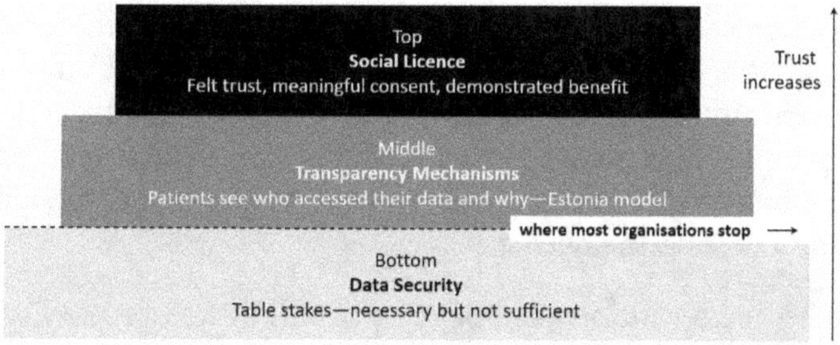

Figure 14. Data security is table stakes—necessary but not sufficient. Transparency mechanisms (the Estonia model) are the middle layer. Social licence—felt trust, meaningful consent, demonstrated benefit—is the goal.

Marc Benioff articulated a related principle at Davos 2026: AI must be grounded in trusted data, woven into existing verified workflows rather than operating as a mysterious external system. This is not just a technical requirement; it is a trust-building strategy. When AI operates within workflows that clinicians and patients already understand, adoption faces less resistance than when AI arrives as an unexplained new layer.

The practical implications are straightforward. Transparency mechanisms should be designed in from the start, not added when patients begin asking questions. Communication about AI should explain not just that it is being used, but why, how and what it means for an individual's care—in language that a retired teacher can understand, not language that satisfies a legal review. Trust is built through demonstrated benefit, not promised benefit. Organisations that can show patients concrete ways their data contributed to better care earn more trust than those making abstract claims about innovation. And control reduces resistance; when patients feel they have meaningful oversight over their data, even if they rarely exercise it, they are substantially more willing to share it.

The organisations building trust infrastructure now will have the social licence to deploy AI at scale. Those treating patient communication as a compliance checkbox will find that no amount of clinical evidence overcomes the absence of felt trust.

Field Lesson 4: Ethics, Safety and the Long View

Yuval Noah Harari offered a sobering perspective at Davos 2026. While most panels focused on quarterly results and five-year plans, he reminded attendees that technological revolutions historically take around two centuries to reach stable states. The Industrial Revolution caused massive social disruption—displacement, exploitation, new forms of poverty alongside new forms of wealth—before societies developed the institutions, regulations and social structures to manage industrial technology responsibly. The first factories existed long before factory safety legislation, labour law or environmental protection. AI is moving faster. The disruption timeline is compressed. Health care sits at the intersection of AI's greatest promise and its greatest risks because the systems being deployed interact with people at their most vulnerable. Harari expressed particular concern about what he described as insufficient attention among leaders to potential social and geopolitical disruption. "You don't need Artificial General Intelligence (AGI) to wreck human systems," he observed. "Extremely primitive AI algorithms in social media have already caused global social disruption." Marc Benioff drew parallel lessons from the early history of social media, arguing that "growth at any cost" had produced measurable harm and that mandatory guardrails for AI were not a constraint on innovation; they were a condition for it being trusted enough to deliver value.

For health care, the implications are direct. AI systems interacting with patients can cause harm through action or inaction. Clinical decision support that misses a diagnosis or recommends an inappropriate treatment has real consequences for real people. Agentic systems that take autonomous action multiply both the potential benefit and the potential harm, and the governance question changes when AI moves from recommending to doing.

Operationalising ethics means moving beyond having a policy to embedding decision points. The question is not "Do we have an AI ethics framework?" but "At what specific points in our AI workflows do ethical considerations get evaluated, by whom and with what authority?" Rather than waiting for perfect ethical consensus before proceeding, which produces either paralysis or uncontrolled deployment, organisations can run bounded experiments with clear governance, learn from what they find and adapt. The liability toolkit from Chapter 3 applies here as it does everywhere in this book: structured experimentation with appropriate oversight, not heroic leaps into the unknown.

Hassabis offered a more measured perspective on the timeline. AI's primary contribution will be to augment human intelligence, and the transition will be gradual enough for society to adapt if organisations invest in that adaptation. But he was explicit about the direction of travel. As AI systems become more autonomous, the stakes of governance failures rise. The governance infrastructure built now will shape outcomes for decades. The organisations taking that seriously will outlast those optimising only for next quarter.

Framework Close: Trust Architecture Assessment

Before your next governance review, work through these questions with your leadership team.

What is your transparency mechanism; can patients see who accessed their data and why? If not, what would it take to build that capability? And if your answer is that legal compliance does not require it, consider whether legal compliance is sufficient for the trust you need to deploy AI at scale. How do you operationalise ethics, not as principles but as decision points? Where in your AI workflows do ethical considerations get evaluated? By whom? How are edge cases escalated, and who has authority to stop a deployment that is causing harm?

What regulatory frameworks are you navigating, and do you have explicit tracking of how they are evolving? Are you building compliance strategies from the most stringent requirements while retaining flexibility for jurisdictions with different approaches?

How do you build trust systematically rather than reactively? What mechanisms exist for patient communication, consent and meaningful control? Are these designed into your AI deployments from the start or added when concerns arise?

For agentic AI specifically, where should AI suggest and wait for human decision? Where does it require explicit approval before acting? Where can it act autonomously within defined guardrails? Have your clinical, legal and technical leaders agreed on these boundaries?

And finally, what is your liability framework for AI-generated harm, and have the relevant leaders aligned on it? The time to answer that question is before an incident, not after.

Organisations that can answer these questions clearly have built trust architecture. Those that cannot are relying on compliance and hoping that is enough.

Back to Samantha

The Pilot Result

Six months later, Samantha presents to the trust's digital governance board.

She has spent those months researching alternatives, building coalitions and drafting proposals. The centrepiece is an Estonia-inspired transparency feature: Patients will be able to see who accessed their records and why. The notifications will not be intrusive—a weekly digest for those who want it, a dashboard showing access patterns over time, real-time alerts available for those who actively opt in.

The resistance was predictable. "Won't patients complain about every access?" "What about emergency situations?" "This creates liability." Samantha had answers for each objection, drawn from the Estonian evidence and adapted to NHS context.

The board approves a pilot.

Three months later, the results surprise nearly everyone. Patient complaints about data access decreased rather than increased. Trust scores improved. And clinicians reported that knowing patients could see their access made them more deliberate about when and why they looked at records—a discipline that had not previously existed.

Samantha calls her mother that evening.

"Remember when you asked who could see your data?"

"I remember," Margaret says. "You didn't know."

"In about 18 months, you'll be able to see for yourself. Everyone who accesses your records. Why they accessed them. When."

There is a long pause.

"That's actually quite reassuring," Margaret says finally. "Knowing I can check even if I never do."

That, Samantha realises, is the whole point. Trust does not require constant verification. It requires the knowledge that verification is possible.

Remember the Five Things

These are not five separate governance requirements. They are a single architecture and an organisation that builds four of them while neglecting the fifth will find the gap undermining everything else.

1. The global regulatory landscape is fragmenting.

   EU, US and Chinese approaches differ fundamentally and are diverging further. The organisations that build adaptive governance now rather than waiting for a clarity that will not arrive will be better positioned as requirements evolve and compliance becomes a differentiator.

2. Trust is built through transparency.

   Estonia's model showed that letting patients see who accessed their data increased willingness to share it. Opacity protects institutions, not patients, and patients know it. Designing transparency in from the start is cheaper and more effective than retrofitting it after trust has been eroded.

3. AI literacy is now a compliance requirement.

   As of February 2025, the EU AI Act requires sufficient AI literacy among staff dealing with AI systems. This is not optional training; it is a legal obligation. And beyond compliance, it is the foundation of governance that actually works, because governance frameworks are only as good as the people implementing them.

4. Agentic AI requires governance frameworks that most organisations have not yet built.

   The shift from recommendation to action changes everything. Where should AI suggest? Where must it wait for human approval? Where can it act within guardrails? Answering these questions before deployment, not after, is what distinguishes responsible innovation from expensive regret.

5. Take the long view seriously.

   The governance infrastructure built now will shape AI outcomes in your organisation for decades. Harari's 200-year frame is not a reason for paralysis; it is a reason for seriousness. The organisations investing in governance as strategic infrastructure will outlast those treating it as compliance overhead.

Chapter 10 asks what you are building toward and what signals, arriving now, deserve your attention before your competitors notice them.

Chapter 10
The Horizon

Preparing for What's Coming Next

Key message: The shift from AI experimentation to industrial execution is happening faster than most health care leaders realise. The organisations preparing now will lead. The rest will spend the next decade catching up. The horizon matters but only if you can see the path from here to there. That path runs through quarterly wins, not transformation announcements.

If You Read Nothing Else, Remember These Five Things

1. Agentic AI is the fundamental shift, and most infrastructure isn't ready for it.

   We're moving from AI that generates text to AI that takes action. From passive systems that respond to prompts to autonomous systems that pursue goals. Health care applications are already emerging: ambient documentation that learns clinician preferences, care coordination agents that chase results and book follow-ups, prior authorisation agents that draft appeals. The technology is moving faster than the platforms underneath it. Chapter 4's operating system thinking isn't optional preparation; it's the prerequisite.

2. Twelve signals deserve your attention through 2027.

   They cluster into four themes: care delivery moving out of clinics (digital GPs, remote pathways, home diagnostics), the agentic shift (commerce, orchestration, big tech entering provision), the physical-AI convergence (robotics, world models, surgical acceleration) and the wildcards (efficiency-first innovation from emerging markets, AI as social connector and at least one breakthrough nobody on any prediction list saw coming). Field Lesson 2 walks each in turn.

3. AGI timeline predictions vary wildly; focus on what you can control.

   Musk says AI will be smarter than any human by late 2026. Amodei says 50% of entry-level white-collar jobs could vanish within five years. Hassabis says the transition will be gradual enough for society to adapt if institutions invest in adaptation. Harari says you don't need AGI to wreck human systems. The practitioner's response to all four: focus on what you can achieve this quarter, not what might happen in five years.

4. Cross-industry learning accelerates health care AI more than benchmarking against other hospitals.

   Finance, logistics, manufacturing and energy are navigating the same scaling, governance and workforce transitions. Visas agentic commerce playbook informs health care coordination. Saudi Aramco's accountability discipline informs health care ROI assessment. The patterns transfer. Health care's traditional insularity is now a liability.

5. The question isn't "What does the future look like?" but "What can we do this quarter?"

   Identify one problem you can solve in six to eight weeks that builds toward the agentic future. Run low-risk experiments. Learn fast. The gap between conference vision and Monday morning reality closes through accumulated small steps, not transformation announcements.

Opening

The Conference

Samantha sits in the back row of a health care leadership conference watching a panel titled "Health Care 2030: The AI-Powered Future." The venue is impressive—a converted warehouse with exposed brick and industrial lighting that signals innovation. The panellists are more impressive still:

CEOs, CMOs, a former health minister, a technology executive whose company is valued at more than most health systems combined.

The predictions are bold. AI doctors handling routine consultations. Robotic surgery performing procedures no human hand could manage. Personalised medicine calibrated to individual genomics. One speaker mentions AGI arriving by late 2027, said with the casual confidence of someone discussing next quarter's earnings.

Samantha thinks of her mother. Margaret still can't get her three specialists to share notes. Last month, the cardiologist prescribed a medication that interacted with what the memory clinic had already prescribed. The pharmacy caught it but only because Samantha had given them a complete medication list from her phone. The systems didn't catch it. The AI didn't catch it. None of the systems on the conference slides existed in her mother's actual care.

The gap between the conference vision and Monday morning reality feels vast enough to induce vertigo.

But then she notices something. The panellists who have actually delivered results—the ones who've scaled AI beyond pilots—talk differently. Less about revolution, more about next steps. Less about transformation, more about the quarter ahead. One speaker, a health care CIO who has actually deployed ambient documentation across 40 hospitals, says something that lands: "Agentic AI is coming. The question isn't whether. It's whether your infrastructure is ready for AI that takes action, not just generates text."

Samantha pulls out her notebook—she still prefers paper for thinking—and starts sketching. Not a vision for 2030. A list of what her trust could realistically achieve in the next two years. Not transformation. Progress.

The horizon matters, she realises. But only if you can see the path from here to there.

Field Lesson 1: The Agentic AI Shift

From Answering to Acting

The most significant AI shift in health care isn't happening in research labs or startup pitches. It's happening in the gap between AI that answers and AI that acts.

Current AI systems are largely passive. They respond to prompts. They generate text, images analysis. They wait for humans to ask questions and then provide answers. This is powerful, but it's not what's coming next.

Agentic AI takes initiative. It pursues goals. It plans multi-step actions and executes them. It adapts when conditions change. It operates more like a junior colleague than a sophisticated search engine. Satya Nadella articulated the evolution at Microsoft as four stages: code completion, where AI finishes what you start; chat assistance, where AI answers questions; agent mode, where AI executes defined tasks and autonomous agents, where AI manages entire workflows. Health care is currently between stages two and three. Stage four is closer than most organisations are ready for.

What's Already Emerging

The practical applications are already operational in pockets. Ambient documentation agents don't just transcribe; they structure encounters, generate summaries, file notes with citations and learn clinician preferences over time. Patient communication agents guide intake, manage reminders and handle rescheduling across web, mobile and phone channels. Prior authorisation agents assemble packets, check policies, reconcile denials and draft appeals. Care coordination agents chase test results, book follow-up appointments and coordinate post-discharge outreach that human staff don't have time to perform.

Transcarent's announcement at CES 2026 captured the shift. Their WayFinding 2.0 platform introduced agentic capabilities that automate scheduling, triage and follow-ups. CEO Glen Tullman framed it bluntly: The chat assistant era is over; the agentic action era has begun. Marketing language aside, the underlying reality is what matters. Autonomous systems are no longer theoretical. They're being deployed.

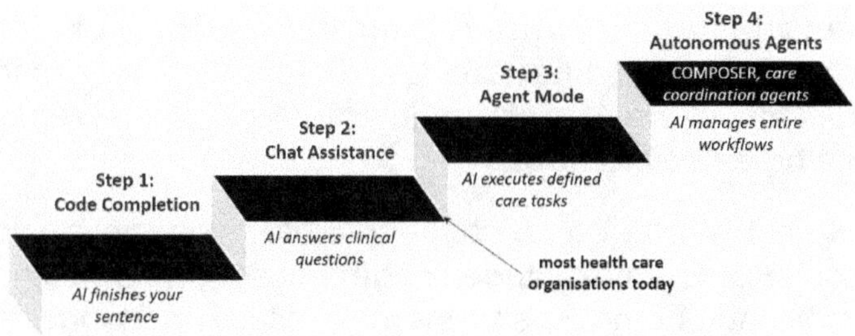

Figure 15. Most health care organisations today sit at Step 2. Step 3 executes defined care tasks. Step 4—COMPOSER, care coordination agents—is already arriving.

UC San Diego's COMPOSER system, discussed in Chapter 6, is the clinical proof. Continuous monitoring of 150 live data points, autonomous prediction of sepsis hours before symptoms appear, autonomous alerting of clinical teams. A 17% reduction in sepsis deaths. That isn't decision support. That's an agent acting to achieve a goal. And it works because the infrastructure beneath it was built for autonomous operation, not retrofitted for it.

The Governance Imperative

When AI only suggests, human oversight is straightforward—clinicians review and decide. When AI takes action autonomously, organisations must define precisely where agents only suggest, where they need human approval and where they can act autonomously within guardrails. Chapter 9's governance architecture isn't preparation for some distant future. It's prerequisite work for systems being deployed now.

Hassabis offered a sobering note worth carrying forward: The next stage is agent-based systems and more autonomous, and the risks scale up alongside the capability. The organisations succeeding with agentic AI take this seriously. They build governance before deployment. They test infrastructure capacity before scaling. They design human-agent collaboration patterns that maintain appropriate oversight without creating bottlenecks that defeat the purpose of automation.

The stepwise journey for most health care organisations runs from today's copilots to task-specific agents, then to process-level agents and eventually to a mesh of agents collaborating across the organisation. Each step requires infrastructure readiness most organisations haven't built. Marc Benioff's vision of the "agentic enterprise"—a unified system where AI orchestrates real-world workflows while humans remain core for values, creativity and relationships—is no longer theoretical. It's being built. The question is whether health care organisations will build it themselves or have it built around them.

Field Lesson 2: Twelve Signals for 2026 – 2027

Prediction is difficult, especially about the future. But pattern recognition across multiple forecasts, Davos discussions and industry analysis reveal signals that deserve attention.

1. Digital GPs for routine care

   AI avatars handling basic health needs—routine consultations, prescription renewals, simple symptom assessment—have moved from speculative to imminent. The question isn't whether this happens but how quickly and who provides it.

2. Agentic commerce in health care

   Visa flagged 2026 as the year agentic commerce moves from concept to deployment—AI agents conducting transactions on behalf of users. The health care parallel: care coordination agents booking appointments, managing medication refills, handling insurance interactions. The administrative friction that defines American health care becomes increasingly automatable.

3. Fully remote outpatient pathways

   Patients completing entire care journeys, from initial consultation through treatment and follow-up, without visiting a physical facility. The pandemic made this imaginable; technology is making it practical.

4. Home-based diagnostics expansion

   Cancer screening, smear tests and other diagnostics moving out of clinics and into homes. Non-invasive blood tests for common cancers may become practical at scale within the next two years. The clinic visit becomes the exception rather than the default.

5. Physical AI and robotics convergence

   Jensen Huang's framing—AI learning "the language of nature", physics, chemistry, biology —converging with robotics. Hassabis's emphasis on systems that understand how the physical world actually works, not just the language people use to describe it. Digital twins at patient, hospital and population levels become operational tools rather than demonstration projects.

6. Big tech care provision

   Not just wearables and apps but actual care delivery. The boundary between the technology company and health care provider continues to blur. Regulatory structures designed for traditional care delivery face strain.

7. AI as a social connector

   Particularly for isolated elderly, AI provides companionship and connection alongside medication reminders. The line between clinical intervention and social support becomes philosophical rather than practical.

8. Efficiency-first innovation

   China's approach—building state-of-the-art models through efficiency rather than scale, using a fraction of the compute resources Western labs assume necessary—challenges the assumption that AI capability requires massive infrastructure investment.

9. World models beyond language

   Hassabis's emphasis from Chapter 5 returns here: systems that understand how reality works, not just how to describe it. Health care applications include predicting how patients will respond to interventions, simulating treatment scenarios and understanding disease progression at a mechanistic level.

10. Remote and robotic surgery acceleration

    AI-assisted procedures with remote capabilities continue to advance. The surgeon in one location, the patient in another, the AI providing real-time guidance to both.

11. Agent sprawl and orchestration

    As organisations deploy multiple agents, coordination becomes critical. Multi-agent systems managing scheduling, clinical support, revenue cycle and patient communication require orchestration layers most organisations haven't designed.

12. At least one breakthrough nobody saw coming

    Think Clustered Regularly Interspaced Short Palindromic Repeats (CRISPR). Think AlphaFold. The unexpected advancement that changes everything. History suggests the developments that change everything are precisely the ones that weren't on anyone's prediction list.

The pattern across these signals is clear: The boundary between health care organisation and technology platform continues to dissolve. Organisations clinging to traditional definitions of their role will find those definitions increasingly irrelevant.

Field Lesson 3: AGI Timeline Realism—A Practitioner's Response

The Range of Predictions

The AGI predictions from technology leaders at Davos 2026 ranged from imminent to cautiously optimistic. Elon Musk projects AI smarter than any individual human by late 2026 or early 2027. Dario Amodei describes a "Moore's Law for intelligence" with three-to-six-month capability leaps and suggests 50% of entry-level white-collar jobs could vanish within five years. Demis Hassabis takes a more measured view; AI's primary role will be to augment human intelligence, and the transition will be gradual enough for society to adapt, provided institutions invest in adaptation. Yuval Harari offered the sharpest counterpoint: You don't need AGI to wreck human systems. Extremely primitive AI algorithms in social media have already caused global social disruption.

For health care practitioners, this divergence creates a strategic challenge. If Musk is right, most current planning horizons are obsolete. If Harari is right, the risk of disruption from current AI is already underestimated. If Hassabis is right, there's time to adapt but only if adaptation starts now.

The Practitioner's Framework

Samantha's response represents the practitioner's perspective: Focus on what you can achieve this quarter, not what might happen in five years. This isn't denial of longer-term possibilities. It's recognition that quarterly wins compound. The organisation that achieves modest improvements every quarter for two years has transformed by the end, even if no single quarter felt like the breakthrough. The organisation waiting for the big breakthrough moment achieves nothing.

The framework runs across four time horizons. For the next quarter, identify one problem you can solve in six to eight weeks that builds toward the agentic future—an ambient documentation pilot, a care coordination agent, a workflow integration test. Small enough to be achievable, significant enough to generate learning. For the next year, close the infrastructure gaps that will block agentic systems: data integration, identity management, governance frameworks for autonomous operation, API architecture that can support agents. None of this is exciting. All of it is essential. For the next two years, build the workforce capabilities that determine whether the technology gets used well: AI literacy across the organisation, the new roles from Chapter 7, training programmes that keep pace with capability evolution. For the uncertain horizon beyond that, build the peer networks that give you visibility into emerging patterns—cross-industry connections, research partnerships, advisory relationships and early warning systems for developments that might affect your strategy.

The gap between conference predictions and Monday morning reality closes through consistent small steps, not transformation announcements. This is the principle the entire book has been building toward.

Field Lesson 4: Building Cross-Industry Peer Networks

The Insularity Trap

Health care has traditionally been insular. Leaders attend conferences, read e-journals and benchmark against health care peers. This insularity used to be defensible; health care's regulatory complexity, clinical specificity and ethical obligations genuinely differ from other industries. It's no longer defensible. The AI challenges facing health care—scaling beyond pilots, governance for autonomous systems, workforce transformation, value measurement—are not unique to the sector. Finance, logistics, manufacturing and energy are navigating remarkably similar transitions.

Visa's journey to agentic commerce offers direct lessons for health care coordination—the same problem of orchestrating actions across systems that don't trust each other with the same need for governance over autonomous behaviour. Saudi Aramco's discipline in measuring AI value across 500 deployments offers lessons for health care ROI assessment that no benchmark can match. Manufacturing's experience with human-robot collaboration offers lessons for augmentation. Financial services' regulatory navigation offers lessons for compliance under fragmenting global frameworks.

The scaling patterns transfer. The governance challenges rhyme. The workforce transformations echo.

Building the Network Deliberately

Cross-industry peer networks don't form by accident. They require intentional effort. Start with close peers—health care leaders facing similar challenges, where the patterns transfer most directly. Then extend deliberately to other industries, finding leaders navigating AI transformation in sectors with different constraints but similar underlying challenges. Look for specific parallels rather than general inspiration: Who has solved a problem you're facing right now? What can you learn from their experience that no health care conference would have surfaced?

The practical next steps fall into five categories:

1. A governance review

   Are your frameworks ready for agentic systems, not just for the passive AI you've deployed so far? The governance designed for systems that suggest won't work for systems that act. Review your decision frameworks now, before you need them.

2. A workforce capability baseline

   Where are the gaps, and what's your AI literacy training plan? The organisations investing in capability now will have adaptable workforces; those waiting will face painful transitions.

3. Opportunity identification

   What's the one problem you could solve in six to eight weeks that builds toward the agentic future? Not a vision exercise. A concrete project with defined scope, measurable outcomes and clear learning objectives.

4. Low-risk experiments

   Ambient documentation pilots, care coordination agents, workflow integration tests. Small enough to be safe, significant enough to generate insight.

5. A contribution commitment

   What will you contribute to collective learning rather than just consume? The field advances when practitioners share honestly. Publish what fails. Share what works. Add to the evidence base that health care AI desperately needs.

The horizon is not a destination to arrive at someday. It's a direction to move toward consistently, starting now.

Framework Close: Horizon Readiness

Before your next strategic planning session, work through these five questions with your leadership team. If you can't answer them clearly, you're hoping the future will wait for you. It won't.

1. Which of the 12 signals are you actively preparing for, and which are you ignoring? Be explicit about priorities and blind spots—the signals you're not tracking are where surprise will come from.
2. Is your infrastructure ready for AI that takes action, not just generates text? If you deployed care coordination agents tomorrow, what would break? Chapter 4's platform thinking isn't optional preparation here. It's the prerequisite.
3. Who are your cross-industry peers, and what can you learn from them this quarter? If the honest answer is "We don't have cross-industry connections", that's the gap to close first.
4. What experiment could you run this quarter that builds toward the horizon? Not a strategic plan. A concrete project with a six-to-eight-week timeline, defined success metrics and a clear learning objective.
5. What will you contribute to collective learning, not just consume? The field needs honest sharing of failures and successes. What will you add?

Back to Samantha

The conference ends. Samantha walks to the train station with her notebook, the list of realistic next steps already organising itself in her mind. The gap between conference vision and Monday morning reality is real. Her mother's specialists still don't share notes. The trust's systems still don't talk to each other. The AI revolution the panellists described feels distant from the daily grind of health care delivery.

But she has learnt something in 20 years of health care leadership: Transformation happens through accumulated small steps, not announced big bangs. The organisations that achieve change are the ones that start with what they can do this quarter and build from there.

She texts her colleague, the clinical informatics lead: "Coffee Monday? Want to discuss ambient documentation pilot."

The response comes immediately: "Finally. Been waiting for someone to ask. 8 am?"

Not AGI by 2027. Not health care revolution by 2030. Just coffee on Monday and a conversation about what they could realistically achieve in the next quarter.

That's how it starts.

Remember The Five Things

These aren't five separate predictions about the future. They're a connected system, and what holds them together is the recognition that the horizon is reached through quarterly discipline, not through five-year vision exercises.

1. Agentic AI is the fundamental shift.

   The infrastructure beneath it is what determines whether organisations lead the transition or get caught flat-footed by it. The platform thinking from Chapter 4, the ontological understanding from Chapter 5, the governance architecture from Chapter 9—these aren't separate chapters. They're the prerequisites for what's arriving now.

2. Twelve signals deserve attention.

   But tracking them only matters if you connect each signal to a specific decision in your current planning cycle. Awareness without action is theatre. Pick the three signals most relevant to your context and decide what they change about your next quarter's priorities.

3. AGI timeline predictions vary.

   The practitioner's response is the same regardless of who turns out to be right. Focus on what you can achieve this quarter. Quarterly wins compound. Five-year visions don't. The organisations transforming health care are the ones executing the discipline repeatedly, not rewriting the playbook every time a new prediction arrives.

4. Cross-industry learning accelerates health care AI.

   The patterns transfer, the challenges rhyme and the workforce transformations echo. Health care's traditional insularity used to be defensible. It isn't any more. The leaders pulling ahead are the ones learning from Visa, Aramco and Microsoft alongside Cleveland Clinic and Kaiser.

5. The question is what you can do this quarter.

   Answering it concretely is the test that separates organisations building toward the horizon from those merely talking about it. One problem. Six to eight weeks. A measurable outcome. Clear learning. That's the discipline. Everything else in this chapter is context for that discipline.

The horizon is visible and the path runs through quarterly wins.

The epilogue follows Samantha two years forward, not to a transformed health care system but to one that has made measurable progress through a thousand small rotations of the flywheel.

Not revolution. Evolution. And perhaps that's the point.

Epilogue
The Flywheel Turns

Samantha's Resolution—Two Years Later

Two years. Not a single transformation moment. A thousand small ones.

The first quarter, they just fixed the data governance. The second, one workflow actually worked. By year one, people stopped asking, “Will this work?” and started asking, “What's next?” The flywheel was turning before anyone declared victory.

The Garden

Samantha sits in her mother's garden. It’s a Tuesday afternoon in early summer, the roses in bloom, the light golden. Margaret naps in the chair beside her, the medication schedule that once required constant vigilance is now managed by systems that actually work.

Margaret’s condition has progressed. That hasn’t changed. Vascular dementia follows its own timeline, indifferent to technological advancement. She has more confused days now than clear ones. The trajectory was never in doubt.

But the system around her has changed. Slowly. Incrementally. Through accumulated small steps that nobody celebrated individually but that compound into something meaningful.

"The trust is finally investing in the boring infrastructure," Samantha told her brother last week. "Patient identifiers that work across systems. Integration that lets the cardiologist see what the memory clinic writes."

"That doesn't sound revolutionary," he said.

"It isn't. That's the point."

And something else—something Samantha pushed for personally. The Estonia-style transparency feature from Chapter 9. Patients can now see exactly who accessed their records and why. The dashboard sits in the patient portal, rarely checked by most people, but its existence changes behaviour. Clinicians know their access is visible. Patients know they could check.

Margaret stirs. "Did I miss the tea?"

"I'll make a fresh pot."

"Before you do..." Margaret's eyes are clearer today, one of her good days. "Show me that thing. The one that shows who looked at my records."

Samantha pulls out her phone and navigates to the portal. "See? Dr Hassan viewed your cardiologist notes yesterday before your appointment. The memory clinic nurse checked your medication list this morning. The pharmacy verified your prescriptions on Friday."

"All those people, keeping track of me." Margaret sounds almost moved.

"All those people, finally able to see each other's work."

"And the robots?" Margaret asks. "The AI you're always talking about?"

Samantha smiles. "Some of it helps. The GP practice uses ambient documentation now. Dr Hassan can look at you while she talks instead of typing. The ED has early warning systems that caught Mrs Patterson's sepsis before it progressed. And we're piloting something new —an AI assistant that handles appointment bookings and chases test results. Small stuff. But it frees up the clinical staff for actual clinical work."

"So the robots are doing the paperwork?"

"The agents are doing the coordination. The humans are doing the caring. That's the point."

Margaret is quiet for a moment. Then: "So it can make health care more human? Like you always hoped?"

"If we choose to build it that way." Samantha pauses, choosing her words carefully. "If we demand evidence over hype. If we build foundations before deploying fancy algorithms. If we keep asking, "Does this help patients, or does it just look impressive?'" She looks at her mother. "That choice isn't automatic. We have to make it, every day."

"You sound tired."

"I am. But also..." Samantha searches for the right word. "Hopeful. Different from two years ago. Back then I felt like I was shouting into a void. Now I feel like we're actually building something."

"Building what?"

"A system that works. Not perfectly. Not everywhere. Not for everything. But better than it was. Measurably better. And getting better still."

The Three Principles, in Action

The three principles that opened this book have become the operating language of how Samantha thinks about her work.

1. Clarity before capability

   She now asks different questions in board meetings. What can we prove, what do we believe, what are we still learning? The framework she introduced in Chapter 8 is now standard for all AI investment proposals at her trust. Others have started asking the same questions. The CFO, once sceptical, now champions honest assessment over optimistic projection.

2. Connection before intelligence

   Her mother's cardiologist can finally see the memory clinic notes. Not through AI magic—through boring integration work that took 18 months and never made it into a board presentation. The Estonia-style transparency feature lets Margaret see who accesses her data. The medication interaction that nearly happened two years ago can't happen now because the systems actually talk to each other. Small victories. Real ones. The kind that don't generate conference presentations but quietly determine whether care is safe.

3. Systems before showcases

   The pilot graveyard is still there—rows of initiatives that launched with fanfare and faded without impact. But new implementations are designed differently. For sustainability, not headlines. The care coordination agent pilot started small and scaled because it worked, not because someone needed a conference slide. The ambient documentation rollout happened practice by practice, learning and adapting as it went. The discipline of asking "What survives when the champion leaves?" has become the discipline of building things built to last.

The Flywheel

Samantha thinks about the flywheel metaphor that's become central to how she explains health care AI transformation.

Two years ago, the flywheel was stuck. Friction everywhere. Poor data quality. Fragmented systems. Clinicians who didn't trust recommendations. Governance structures that paralysed rather than enabled. The first push was the hardest. Fixing data governance felt like pushing against immovable resistance. No visible progress for months.

Then, slowly, the wheel began to turn. Clinician adoption improved because recommendations actually made sense. Better adoption generated better data. Better data improved AI performance. Better performance built trust. Trust enabled more data sharing. Each rotation reinforced the next.

The flywheel isn't spinning freely yet. There's still friction. There are still stuck points. But it's moving. And each rotation gets easier than the last.

That's transformation. Not a dramatic moment of revelation. A thousand small rotations, each building on the last, momentum accumulating until the system's own dynamics take over from organisational effort.

The Invitation

You now have what you need.

Clarity about AI's reality in health care, the gap between promise and delivery and the uncomfortable truths that create decision clarity. Vocabulary to decode vendor claims and evaluate evidence honestly. Understanding of where implementations fail and how they succeed.

Recognition that transformation requires infrastructure, not just algorithms. Awareness that agentic AI is arriving and so are the governance frameworks to prepare for it. Tools to assess value honestly, build trust systematically and prepare for a horizon that's approaching faster than most leaders realise.

What you do with this knowledge is up to you.

The core message remains what it was in the introduction: Demand evidence, build foundations, keep humans central. Clarity before capability. Connection before intelligence. Systems before showcases.

If you've found value in these pages, don't just consume; contribute. Share what works in your organisation. Publish what fails. Add to the evidence base that health care AI desperately needs. Build the peer networks that accelerate learning. The field advances when practitioners share honestly, not when vendors control the narrative.

The First Push

Margaret has fallen asleep again in the garden chair. Samantha watches her mother breathe, the familiar rhythm unchanged from childhood, and thinks about what health care could become.

Not the conference vision of AI doctors and robotic surgery and personalised medicine calibrated to individual genomics. That future may come, or it may not. It's not the future she can control.

What she can control: the next quarterly win. The next small step. The next rotation of the flywheel.

Monday morning, she'll walk into the trust and face the same challenges she faced two years ago, with the same constraints and the same resistant systems and the same gap between what's promised and what's delivered.

But the flywheel is turning now. And that changes everything.

The flywheel is waiting. What's your first push?

About the Author

Janahan Tharmaratnam has spent two decades implementing AI and digital transformation across some of the world's most demanding health systems—the National Health Service in the UK, the modernising Gulf states of the United Arab Emirates, Saudi Arabia and Qatar and large North American academic medical centres. He has worked with ministries of health, sovereign wealth funds and hospital boards on the operating model changes that determine whether AI succeeds at scale or fails in pilot.

A frequent contributor to industry forums on healthcare AI, including the World Economic Forum at Davos, World Health Organization and the HIMSS Expert Forums, his focus is the gap between AI and technology promise and frontline reality.

He lives in the United Arab Emirates with his family. Healthcare NEXT is his first book.

About PublishU

PublishU enables you to tell your story or communicate your message by writing and publishing a book worldwide.

"I never thought I would be able to write a book, let alone in 100 days... now I'm asking what else have I told myself that I can't do that I actually can?"'

PublishU Author

To find out more visit

www.PublishU.com

Endnotes

1. Daneshjou, R. et al. Disparities in dermatology AI performance on a diverse, curated clinical image set. Science Advances, 8(31), 2022. DOI: 10.1126/sciadv.abq6147.

2. Rezk E, Eltorki M, El-Dakhakhni W. Improving Skin Color Diversity in Cancer Detection: Deep Learning Approach. JMIR Dermatology. 2022;5(3):e39143. DOI: 10.2196/39143.

3. Daneshjou, R. et al. Disparities in dermatology AI performance on a diverse, curated clinical image set. Science Advances, 8(31), 2022. DOI: 10.1126/sciadv.abq6147.

4. Muralidharan, V. et al. A scoping review of reporting gaps in FDA-approved AI medical devices. npj Digital Medicine, 7, 2024. DOI: 10.1038/s41746-024-01270-x; Callahan, A. et al. How AI is used in FDA-authorized medical devices: a taxonomy across 1,016 authorizations. npj Digital Medicine, 2025. DOI: 10.1038/s41746-025-01800-1.

5. Daneshjou, R. et al. Disparities in dermatology AI performance on a diverse, curated clinical image set. Science Advances, 8(31), 2022. DOI: 10.1126/sciadv.abq6147.

6. Muralidharan, V. et al. A scoping review of reporting gaps in FDA-approved AI medical devices. npj Digital Medicine, 7, 2024. DOI: 10.1038/s41746-024-01270-x; Callahan, A. et al. How AI is used in FDA-authorized medical devices: a taxonomy across 1,016 authorizations. npj Digital Medicine, 2025. DOI: 10.1038/s41746-025-01800-1.

7. Olson KD, Meeker D, Troup M, Barker TD, Nguyen VH, Manders JB, Stults CD, Jones VG, Shah SD, Shah T, Schwamm LH. Use of Ambient AI Scribes to Reduce Administrative Burden and Professional Burnout. JAMA Network Open. 2025;8(10):e2534976. DOI: 10.1001/jamanetworkopen.2025.34976.

8. Stults CD, Martinez MC, Szwerinski NK, Rabbani N, Jones VG, et al. Evaluation of an Ambient Artificial Intelligence Documentation Platform for Clinicians. JAMA Network Open. 2025;8(5):e2510144. DOI: 10.1001/jamanetworkopen.2025.10144.

9. Peterson Health Technology Institute (PHTI). Adoption of AI in Healthcare Delivery Systems: Early Applications and Impacts. PHTI Report, March 2025. Available at https://phti.org/assessment/adoption-of-ai-in-healthcare-delivery-systems-early-applications-impacts/.

10. Boussina, A., Shashikumar, S.P., Malhotra, A. et al. Impact of a deep learning sepsis prediction model on quality of care and survival. npj Digital Medicine, 7(14), 2024. DOI: 10.1038/s41746-023-00986-6.

www.ingramcontent.com/pod-product-compliance
Lightning Source LLC
La Vergne TN
LVHW022159200926
848481LV00006B/1787